Sports Nutrition
Workbook and Assessments

Heather Hedrick Fink, MS, RD, CSSD
Assistant Director of Educational Services
National Institute for Fitness and Sport
Indianapolis, Indiana

Lisa A. Burgoon, MS, RD, CSSD, LDN
Sports Dietitian and Visiting Teaching Associate
Department of Food Science and Human Nutrition
University of Illinois
Urbana-Champaign, Illinois

Alan E. Mikesky, PhD, FACSM
Professor
School of Physical Education and Tourism Management
Indiana University-Purdue University
Indianapolis, Indiana

D1604602

JONES AND BARTLETT PUBLISHERS
Sudbury, Massachusetts
BOSTON   TORONTO   LONDON   SINGAPORE

World Headquarters
Jones and Bartlett Publishers
40 Tall Pine Drive
Sudbury, MA 01776
978-443-5000
info@jbpub.com
www.jbpub.com

Jones and Bartlett Publishers Canada
6339 Ormindale Way
Mississauga, Ontario L5V 1J2
Canada

Jones and Bartlett Publishers International
Barb House, Barb Mews
London W6 7PA
United Kingdom

Jones and Bartlett's books and products are available through most bookstores and online booksellers. To contact Jones and Bartlett Publishers directly, call 800-832-0034, fax 978-443-8000, or visit our website, www.jbpub.com.

Production Credits
Acquisitions Editor: Shoshanna Goldberg
Senior Associate Editor: Amy L. Bloom
Editorial Assistant: Kyle Hoover
Production Manager: Julie Champagne Bolduc
Production Assistant: Jessica Steele Newfell
Associate Marketing Manager: Jody Sullivan
V.P., Manufacturing and Inventory Control: Therese Connell
Composition: Publishers' Design and Production Services
Cover Design: Scott Moden
Cover Image: © Jones and Bartlett Publishers. Photographed by Kimberly Potvin
Printing and Binding: Courier Stoughton
Cover Printing: Courier Stoughton

ISBN 978-0-7637-6194-3

6048

Printed in the United States of America

13 12 11 10 09   10 9 8 7 6 5 4 3 2 1

Contents

Preface

Mastering a new sport skill requires practice and so does learning new information. Practice through repetition is the key to success. Although the textbook, *Practical Applications in Sports Nutrition, Second Edition*, includes various ways of helping students apply the information provided in each chapter to their daily lives (e.g., case studies and study questions), we developed this workbook to serve two main purposes:

1. To provide the student with expanded and alternative activities that will foster the use of information provided in each chapter of the main text

2. To provide the instructor with challenging chapter-specific activities that can be used to evaluate student progress

This workbook is intended to serve as a companion to the *Second Edition* of *Practical Applications in Sports Nutrition* to provide students with additional practice opportunities using real-life examples, problems, and case studies. Crossword puzzles also are included in each chapter to help students become more comfortable with the key terms encountered by sport nutrition professionals. The more times the terms and concepts presented in the chapters are practiced, the greater the odds that the information will be mastered.

The chapters in this workbook parallel the chapters in the main text. The goal is to challenge students in a variety of creative ways, giving them opportunities to practice what they have learned in the classroom and from the readings in the main text. The ultimate goal of the realistic scenarios and critical thinking questions in this workbook is to give students a better perspective as to why they need to invest the time and effort necessary to master the information.

Answers are not provided in the student workbook for several reasons. First, we eliminate the urge to simply turn to the answer section without first consulting the main text to research the information needed to answer the case studies or questions. Second, the instructor is provided an opportunity to give students the answers after they have engaged in inquisitive exploration or to use the workbook activities as graded assignments. Regardless, successful completion of the activities in each chapter of this workbook requires inquisitive exploration. Students are encouraged to refer back to *Practical Applications in Sports Nutrition, Second Edition*, and to read specific sections with the intent of finding the answers to the problems, case studies, or crossword puzzles. This type of directed, purposeful reading has been shown in the pedagogical literature to be effective in helping students learn.

We hope that both students and instructors find the activities in this workbook challenging, enjoyable, and beneficial.

Heather Fink, Lisa Burgoon, and Alan Mikesky

Authors of *Practical Applications in Sports Nutrition, Second Edition*

Name: _____ Course Number: _____

Section: _____ Date: _____

CHAPTER 1

Introduction to Sports Nutrition

MyPyramid Diet and Physical Activity Assessment

Part 1: Analysis of Diet

The first assessment of your diet will be to compare your food intake to the recommended amounts from each of the food groups on MyPyramid. This will give you a good idea of how well your diet meets the nutrition principles of variety, balance, and moderation. MyPyramid emphasizes three key messages:

- Make smart choices from every food group
- Find your balance between food and physical activity
- Get the most nutrition out of your calories

MyPyramid is pictured on page 2. This graphic represents a personalized approach to healthy eating and physical activity. To view a color graphic, go to the MyPyramid Web site, http://www.mypyramid.gov. Variety is represented by the six color bands, which represent the five food groups of MyPyramid as well as oils. Moderation is represented by the narrowing of each food group band from bottom to top, with the wider base for foods with little or no solid fats or added sugars to be selected more often than foods with more fat and sugar found at the top. Proportionality is shown by the different widths of the food group bands. The widths suggest how much food a person should choose from each group. Activity is represented by the person climbing the steps. The slogan "Steps to a Healthier You" encourages gradual improvement by taking small steps to improve your diet and lifestyle each day.

To begin your assessment, go to the MyPyramid Web site, http://www.mypyramid .gov. You will be asked to enter your age, sex, and activity level. To determine your activity level, refer to your activity records, and add up the minutes of moderate, vigorous, or strenuous activity you do daily that is in addition to your normal daily routine. You will have three options of activity levels: less than 30 minutes, 30–60 minutes, and more than 60 minutes. Entering this data will result in your own MyPyramid Plan listing the recommended amounts of food from each food group, amount of fats and oils, and amount of discretionary calories. This is based on one of 12 calorie patterns. Print out a PDF version of your results.

To compare your daily food intake with your recommended intake in each of the MyPyramid food groups, you will use the online MyPyramid Tracker and click on the "Assess Food Intake" icon. First, record your daily intake of amount and types of food eaten on the *MyPyramid Diet Analysis* form on page 3. Use a separate form for each day you will analyze. Using the food intake data on these forms, follow the online instructions to enter the data into the Tracker program. Enter each 24-hour diet log separately into MyPyramid

MyPyramid

MyPyramid.gov

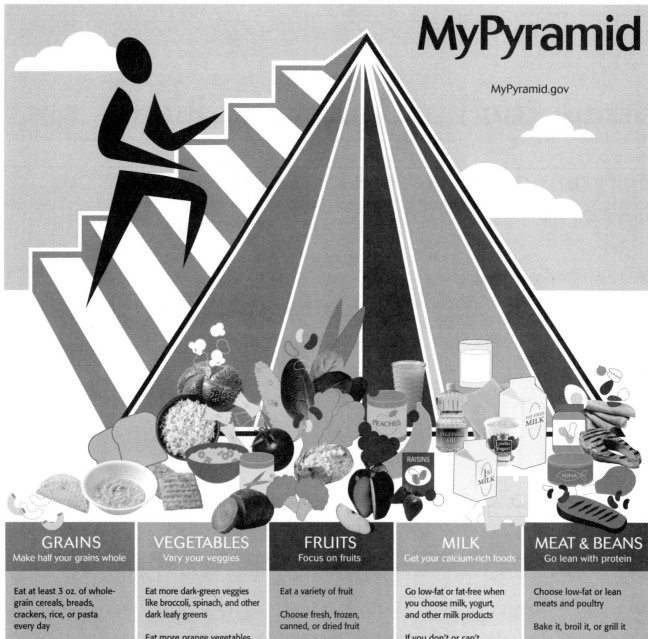

GRAINS
Make half your grains whole

VEGETABLES
Vary your veggies

FRUITS
Focus on fruits

MILK
Get your calcium-rich foods

MEAT & BEANS
Go lean with protein

GRAINS	VEGETABLES	FRUITS	MILK	MEAT & BEANS
Eat at least 3 oz. of whole-grain cereals, breads, crackers, rice, or pasta every day 1 oz. is about 1 slice of bread, about 1 cup of breakfast cereal, or 1/2 cup of cooked rice, cereal, or pasta	Eat more dark-green veggies like broccoli, spinach, and other dark leafy greens Eat more orange vegetables like carrots and sweetpotatoes Eat more dry beans and peas like pinto beans, kidney beans, and lentils	Eat a variety of fruit Choose fresh, frozen, canned, or dried fruit Go easy on fruit juices	Go low-fat or fat-free when you choose milk, yogurt, and other milk products If you don't or can't consume milk, choose lactose-free products or other calcium sources such as fortified foods and beverages	Choose low-fat or lean meats and poultry Bake it, broil it, or grill it Vary your protein routine — choose more fish, beans, peas, nuts, and seeds

For a 2,000-calorie diet, you need the amounts below from each food group. To find the amounts that are right for you, go to MyPyramid.gov.

Eat 6 oz. every day	Eat 2 1/2 cups every day	Eat 2 cups every day	Get 3 cups every day; for kids aged 2 to 8, it's 2	Eat 5 1/2 oz. every day

Find your balance between food and physical activity
- Be sure to stay within your daily calorie needs.
- Be physically active for at least 30 minutes most days of the week.
- About 60 minutes a day of physical activity may be needed to prevent weight gain.
- For sustaining weight loss, at least 60 to 90 minutes a day of physical activity may be required.
- Children and teenagers should be physically active for 60 minutes every day, or most days.

Know the limits on fats, sugars, and salt (sodium)
- Make most of your fat sources from fish, nuts, and vegetable oils.
- Limit solid fats like butter, margarine, shortening, and lard, as well as foods that contain these.
- Check the Nutrition Facts label to keep saturated fats, *trans* fats, and sodium low.
- Choose food and beverages low in added sugars. Added sugars contribute calories with few, if any, nutrients.

MyPyramid Diet and Physical Activity Assessment

Tracker, and click on "save and analyze." You will use these analyses to compare your intake to the recommended guidelines from MyPyramid, the Dietary Guidelines for Americans, and in comparing energy intake and energy expenditure.

MyPyramid Diet Analysis

My Intake:	Amount Eaten in Food Groups (ounce or cup equivalents)						
Food or Beverage	Grains (oz-equiv)	Vegetable (cups)	Fruit (cups)	Milk (cups)	Meat (oz-equiv)	Oils (tsp)	Discretionary Calories

After you have clicked "save and analyze," select and analyze both the "Meeting the 2005 Dietary Guidelines" and the "MyPyramid Recommendation" analyses. Print both of these analyses and use them to complete the assignment.

The table below lists suggested amounts of food to consume from the five basic food groups and oils to meet recommended nutrition intakes at 12 different calorie levels for adults and children over the age of 2. There are no food intake pattern calorie levels for adults below 1,600 calories. For young adults ages 19–30, the calorie range for females is 2,000–2,400, and the calorie range for males is 2,400–3,000, depending on activity level. Nutrient and energy contributions from each group are calculated according to the nutrient-dense forms of foods in each group (e.g., lean meats and fat-free milk). The table also shows the discretionary calorie allowance[7] that can be accommodated within each calorie level.

	Daily Amount of Food from Each Group											
Calorie Level	1,000	1,200	1,400	1,600	1,800	2,000	2,200	2,400	2,600	2,800	3,000	3,200
Fruits[1] (in cups/day)	1	1	1.5	1.5	1.5	2	2	2	2	2.5	2.5	2.5
Vegetables[2] (in cups/day)	1	1.5	1.5	2	2.5	2.5	3	3	3.5	3.5	4	4
Grains[3] (in ounce-equivalents/day)	3	4	5	5	6	6	7	8	9	10	10	10
Meat and Beans[4] (in ounce-equivalents/day)	2	3	4	5	5	5.5	6	6.5	6.5	7	7	7
Milk[5] (in cups/day)	2	2	2	3	3	3	3	3	3	3	3	3
Oils[6] (in teaspoons/day)	3	4	4	5	5	6	6	7	8	8	10	11
Discretionary Calorie Allowance[7] (total remaining calories)	165	171	171	132	195	267	290	362	410	426	512	648

Footnotes

1. The Fruit Group includes all fresh, frozen, canned, and dried fruits and fruit juices.

2. The Vegetable Group includes all fresh, frozen, canned, and fried vegetables and vegetable juices. Five vegetables subgroups are recommended each week:

Dark green vegetables	(3 cups/week)
Orange vegetables	(2–2.5 cups/week)
Legumes	(3–3.5 cups/week)
Starchy vegetables	(3–9 cups/week)
Other vegetables	(6.5–10 cups/week)

    For your recommended amounts from each subgroup, refer to the MyPyramid Plan you calculated at http://www.mypyramid.gov.

3. The Grains Group includes all foods made from wheat, rice, oats, cornmeal, and barley, such as bread, pasta, oatmeal, breakfast cereals, tortillas, and grits. At least half of all grains consumed should be whole grains.

4. The Meat and Beans Group includes meat, poultry, fish, eggs, nuts, nut butters, legumes (cooked dry beans), tofu, and seeds.

5. The Milk Group includes all fluid milk products and foods made from milk, such as yogurt and cheese.

6. Oils include fats that are liquid at room temperature and are from some fish and many different plants, such as canola, corn, olive, soybean, and sunflower. Some foods are naturally high in oils, like nuts, olives, some fish, and avocados. Foods that are mainly oil include mayonnaise, certain salad dressings, and soft margarine.

7. The discretionary calorie allowance is the amount of calories remaining after accounting for the calories needed for all food groups (using only foods that are fat-free or low-fat with no added sugars) and oils. It allows you to select higher fat and sugar options from the food groups, as well as "extras." For more information, go to "Inside the Pyramid" and then click on "Discretionary Calories" at the MyPyramid Web site.

MyPyramid Analysis

Using your MyPyramid Plan PDF and printouts from each day of MyPyramid Recommendation analyses, complete the *Total Daily Amount Eaten in MyPyramid Food Groups* chart below. Take the average of each of the food groups and discretionary calories columns, and compare these to the PDF printout for your MyPyramid Plan. Identify the areas of shortage and surplus on the chart.

Total Daily Amount Eaten in MyPyramid Food Groups							
	Grains (oz-equiv)	Vegetable (cups)	Fruit (cups)	Milk (cups)	Meat (oz-equiv)	Oils (tsp)	Discretionary Calories
Day One							
Day Two							
Day Three							
Day Four							
Day Five							
Day Six							
Day Seven							
Average (Total ÷ # of Days)							
Recommended (Refer to your MyPyramid Plan)							
Shortage							
Surplus							

What is the recommended calorie intake level on your MyPyramid Plan?

_____

List the food groups in which you met the recommended amount of food on most days:

_____

List the food groups in which you consumed less than the recommended amount of food on most days:

_____

List the food groups in which you consumed more than the recommended amount of food on most days:

_____

Dietary Guidelines Analysis

Review the printouts from each day of the Dietary Guidelines Recommendations analyses. The emoticon for each category tells you how your diet compares to these recommendations.

List the Dietary Guidelines categories in which you met the recommendations on most days:

_____

List the Dietary Guidelines categories in which you did not meet the recommendations on most days:

_____

In the Dietary Guidelines categories in which you did not meet the recommendations, list the categories that you:

Consumed more than the amount recommended:

_____

Consumed less than the amount recommended:

_____

Select one area from the Dietary Guideline analysis in which you did not completely meet the recommendation. List specific foods and amounts of foods that you should consume on a daily basis to improve your dietary intake in this category.

Think about both parts of the dietary assessment: MyPyramid and Dietary Guidelines recommendations. What dietary changes do you need to make in order to meet both sets of guidelines?

Why is it important to meet these guidelines?

How are both sets of guidelines similar? How are they different? How can they be used together to help individuals improve or maintain health?

Select one day of those you analyzed, and create a revised menu for that day. Turn in the original and the revised menu along with an explanation of how the revised menu meets more of the recommended nutrition guidelines.

Part 2: Analysis of Physical Activity

Getting adequate physical activity is an important part of staying healthy. You will use the MyPyramid Tracker to assess your physical activity level, and then compare it to recommended levels and to your dietary intake. To complete this part of the assignment, go to MyPyramid Tracker and click on the "Assess Your Physical Activity" icon. It may be easiest to first record some or all of your physical activities on the *Physical Activity Log* on page 8. Record each of your physical activities in minutes for one 24-hour (1,440-minute) period. Follow the online instructions to enter activity data into the Tracker system. When you are finished recording all 1,440 minutes, click on "Save and Analyze," and then click on "Physical Activity Analysis." Print this summary report. Enter the data from the report onto the *Total Daily Physical Activity* table on page 9, and enter the calorie level you listed from your MyPyramid Plan in Part 1.

Physical Activity Log

Sample Physical Activity Log
Record all activities in one 24-hour (1,440 minute) period.

Activity	Minutes	Intensity Level
Sleeping	420	n/a
Sitting in class, taking notes	300	n/a
Running	45	8 min/mile pace
Watching television	75	n/a
Walking to class	40	Leisurely pace
Walking to class	20	Fast
Eating	50	n/a
Cooking/food preparation	35	n/a

Blank Physical Activity Log

Record all activities in one 24-hour (1,440-minute) period.

Activity	Minutes	Intensity Level

MyPyramid Diet and Physical Activity Assessment

Total Daily Physical Activity

Credited Minutes	
Total calories expended from physical activity	
Physical activity score (out of 100)	
Physical activity assessment	
List two activities with highest calorie expenditure	
List two activities with lowest calorie expenditure	
Calorie level listed on your MyPyramid Plan diet	

Describe what your physical activity score means.

How do your calorie expenditure and calorie intake recommendation levels compare?

What is your weight goal (i.e., weight loss, weight gain, or weight maintenance)?

Based on your answer to how your calorie expenditure and intake compare, as well as your weight goal, discuss how you could modify your diet and/or exercise level to achieve your goal.

Reading Food Labels

Directions: Go to your local grocery store and buy a can of Campbell's Chunky Soup. Using a sharp knife, slice downward along the right edge of the Nutrition Facts panel so that you can peel the entire label off of the can without damaging it. Answer each of the following questions. For questions a–e below, circle the location of where you found the information on the label using a permanent marker. Staple the label to the worksheet.

a. What is the net weight of the contents?

b. Which three ingredients in the soup are most abundant based on weight?

    1. _____

    2. _____

    3. _____

c. Where is the Campbell Soup Company located?

d. How many servings are in the can?

e. How many grams of protein are provided per serving?

f. How many grams of carbohydrates are provided in the entire can?

g. What is the percentage of calories from fat?

h. Is the soup you bought within the recommended percentage range for fat consumption?

i. How many grams of trans fats are in one serving of the soup?

j. What is the total amount of sodium in the entire can?

k. If you consumed the entire can for a meal, would you consider the sodium content to be high?

Explain why or why not: _____

_____

_____

_____

_____

_____

_____

You Are the Nutrition Coach

Please read each case study listed below, and answer the associated questions.

1. During a presentation to a group of high school football players and coaches, you mention that the MyPyramid Web site is an excellent resource for athletes. One of the assistant coaches interjects and states that the MyPyramid food guidance system is too basic and not applicable for the needs of teenage football players.

   Question: How would you respond to this comment?

2. Kelly is a 35-year-old lawyer. She has been exercising regularly for 2 years. She schedules an appointment with you to discuss quick and easy meal planning ideas. Kelly works 50 hours per week, commutes 60 minutes roundtrip, and exercises 1–2 hours daily. She complains that she is too tired to cook a meal when she arrives at home, and therefore, typically microwaves a pizza, burrito, or veggie burger for dinner. Currently, she is consuming only 1–2 servings of fruits and vegetables per day because "they take too long to prepare."

   Question: Using the Dietary Guidelines for Americans, what recommendations would you provide to Kelly?

3. During your initial consultation with a client, you inquire about his fruit preferences. He replies that he enjoys fresh, canned, and dried fruits, but avoids juices because "they have too much sugar."

   Question: How would you respond to this comment? Include in your answer suggestions for interpreting the nutrition information provided on a container of fruit juice.

Crossword Puzzle

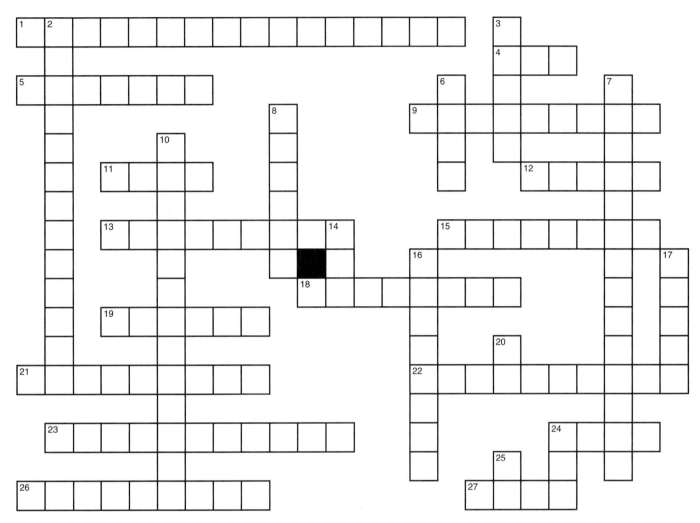

Across

1. the Dietary Guidelines for Americans also recommends this (2 words)
4. the body's direct source of energy (abbrev.)
5. less than 0.5 g of fat per serving (2 words)
9. nutrients that cannot be made by the body
11. one micronutrient required to appear on food labels
12. prefix used to describe nutrients, like vitamins and minerals
13. the "E" in EAR
15. these exist in water and fat soluble forms
18. sodium, iodine, calcium, and phosphorus, to name a few
19. food label ingredients are listed in order based on this
21. a food guide for healthy eating
22. adding nutrients lost in processing back to foods
23. the Nutrition Facts panel information on food labels is based on this (2 words)
24. nutrient category with the highest energy density
26. a skill that sports nutrition professionals must develop and practice
27. congressional legislation that requires food labeling (abbrev.)

Down

2. developing a good sport nutrition plan starts with this (2 words)
3. most abundant, nonenergy yielding nutrient in the body
6. overseer of the Dietary Guidelines for Americans (abbrev.)
7. carbohydrates, fats, and proteins
8. a type of claim found on food labels
10. addition of "foreign" nutrients to foods
14. newer, expanded version of RDA (abbrev.)
16. composed of amino acids
17. specialty area in nutrition for active individuals and athletes
20. this is used when an RDA has not been established (abbrev.)
24. food safety agency (abbrev.)
25. intakes above this increase risk for toxicity (abbrev.)

Name: _____   Course Number: _____

Section: _____   Date: _____

CHAPTER 2

Nutrients: Ingestion to Energy Metabolism

Digestion

Using the list of words below, place the correct term in the blank provided.

lipoprotein   vitamins   carbohydrate   glucose
water   minerals   small intestine   galactose
fructose   triglyceride   free fatty acid   GluT
amino acid pool   gall bladder   stomach   large intestine
amylase

1. Digestion of this nutrient begins in the mouth. _____

2. Mehanical churning of food occurs in this pouch-like portion of the digestive tract. _____

3. Most absorption of nutrients takes place here. _____

4. This sac-like structure secretes bile to aid in fat digestion. _____

5. Specialized membrane glucose carrier proteins. _____

6. Bacteria acts on undigested food in this portion of the digestive tract. _____

7. This enzyme breaks down starch in the mouth. _____

8. This nutrient passes across cell membranes using passive diffusion. _____

9. These monosaccharides require active transport to diffuse across cell membranes. _____

10. This monosaccharide uses facilitated diffusion to pass through cell membranes. _____

11. A lipid that contains a glycerol with three attached fatty acids. _____

12. The name for the fatty acids once they are cleaved off the glycerol. _____

13. A lipid compound that carries triglycerides through the intestinal cells. _____

14. A collection of amino acids found in body fluids and tissues. _____

15. These molecules do not require breakdown into smaller units for absorption. _____

Energy Metabolism

1. During a 3-minute boxing round, identify which energy system(s) is being used at the times listed below:

   _____ First punch within 3 seconds of starting the round

   _____ A continuous flurry of jabs and fast moves lasting about 45 seconds after 1.5 minutes into the round

   _____ Right at the end of 3 minutes, while moving around the ring

   _____ During the 1-minute rest between rounds

2. For each of the energy systems you listed above, list which macronutrient(s) is being utilized.

   _____ First punch within 3 seconds of starting the round

   _____ A continuous flurry of jabs and fast moves lasting about 45 seconds after 1.5 minutes into the round

   _____ Right at the end of 3 minutes, while moving around the ring

   _____ During the 1-minute rest between rounds

3. Carefully read the following sentences, as they apply to the bioenergetics occurring in an athlete's leg muscles during the *first 3 minutes* of the race. Circle the word or words in the sentences that are incorrect. Write the correct word or words in the margin. Clearly indicate which words are being replaced with your suggestions.

Carrie is standing at the starting line awaiting the starter's gun to begin the Indianapolis Half Marathon. In the initial 5 seconds as she begins to accelerate to race pace, the 4 energy systems begin to respond to the increased need for energy. The immediate ATP needs are met initially by the muscle's existing stores of ATP and lactic acid, which constitute what is known as the muscle cell's anaerobic energy system. Almost as quickly, the phosphagen energy system begins metabolizing fats for energy, and starts to contribute towards the increased need for ATP. About 2 minutes into the race, the aerobic energy system has had time to ramp up its production of creatine phosphate, and begins to produce all of the energy Carrie's muscles need. Fats and proteins are the primary macronutrients metabolized by the aerobic energy system during the race. The other 3 energy systems back off and play only a minor role in supplying the needed ATP from then on.

You Are the Nutrition Coach

Please read each case study listed below, and answer the associated questions.

1. You are a glucose molecule in a disaccharide found in a drink that was sipped by an athlete who is about to begin running a 1600m (1 mile) race. Put the words in the list below in the appropriate order to describe the process of your journey from the mouth and ultimately to the muscle cells for energy.

   Word list:

   electron transport system

   active transport

   stomach

   pyruvate

   brush border disaccharidases

   carbon dioxide and water

   mouth

   citric acid cycle

   glucose transporters

   duodenum

   glycolysis

   jejunum

   blood

   esophagus

2. During a consultation with Tommy, a high school freshman soccer player, he asks you what he should eat for breakfast before hard morning practices. He sleeps until 6:00 AM and has 1 hour before practice begins at 7:00 AM.

   Question: What breakfast ideas would you recommend to Tommy? Be specific with types and amounts of food and beverages, and explain why you are suggesting these meals.

Name: _____   Course Number: _____

Section: _____   Date: _____

Crossword Puzzle

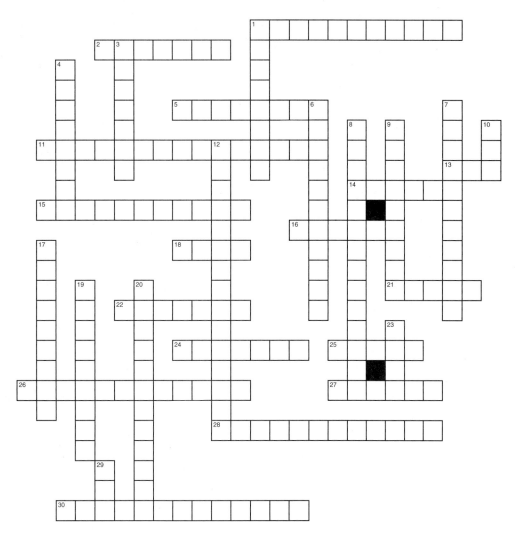

Across

1. fatty stools
2. individuals who cannot digest dairy products are deficient of this
5. section of the GI tract where digestive enzymes from the pancreas are released
11. all carbohydrates are made up of these
13. fat enzyme that lines capillary walls in muscle and adipose tissue (abbrev.)
14. fatty acids belong to this group of compounds
15. a form of absorption involving cell membrane internalization
16. moistens and softens foods put into the mouth
18. fatty acids not attached to glycerol are this
21. fatty acid chains of < 4 carbons are considered this
22. a type of lipase found in saliva
24. type of diffusion that does not require a transporter or energy
25. these structures increase the surface area of the intestinal walls
26. the unfolding or loss of shape of proteins during digestion
27. feces storage site within the gastrointestinal tract
28. a glycerol molecule with three fatty acids attached
30. the process of copying genetic material in the cell nucleus

Down

1. duodenal hormone important in fatty acid digestion
3. carbohydrate-digesting enzyme found in saliva
4. form of carbohydrates in human cells
6. the process of chewing
7. that break fats into very small globules
8. makes up the majority of the gastrointestinal tract (2 words)
9. attaches the oral cavity to the stomach
10. responsible for the denaturation of proteins in the stomach (abbrev.)
12. form of absorption that requires energy and protein carriers (2 words)
17. cellular organelles that build proteins
19. lack of just one of these can prevent formation of a protein (2 words)
20. fat carrier molecules found in the blood
23. glucose transporter (abbrev.)
29. genes are made up of this (abbrev.)

Crossword Puzzle

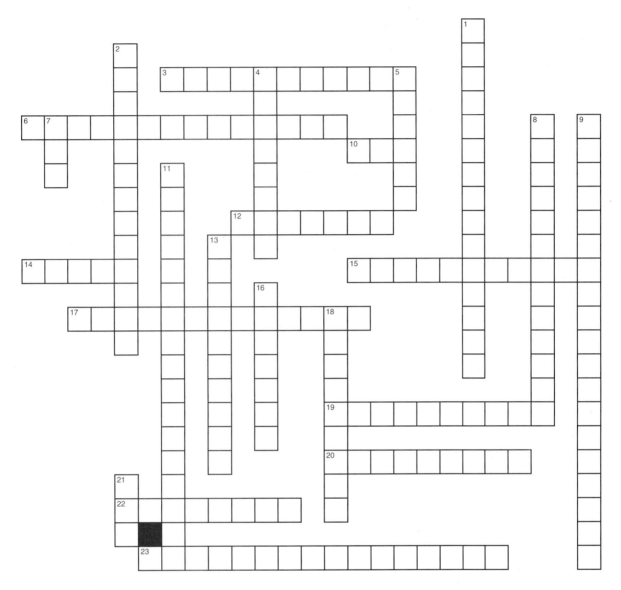

Across

3. a unit of measure for energy
6. the energy nutrients
10. the minimal amount of energy needed to keep the body alive (abbrev.)
12. the inability to maintain performance at a given level
14. one of the end products of aerobic metabolism
15. process of removing the nitrogen component from amino acids
17. the study of how energy is captured, transferred, and utilized in cells
19. the energy system also known as the immediate energy system
20. the energy system that forms lactic acid
22. an energy-requiring process that forms more complex molecules
23. a sequence of chemical reactions (2 words)

Down

1. the process of making glucose from proteins
2. the aerobic powerhouse of cells
4. the form of energy humans rely on for survival
5. has no describable features or mass but provides for cellular work
7. adenosine molecule with two phosphates attached to it (abbrev.)
8. first metabolic pathway in the breakdown of fatty acids (2 words)
9. energy supplement used by sprint athletes (2 words)
11. immediate, high-energy compound other than ATP (2 words)
13. an aerobic metabolic pathway common to all macronutrients (2 words)
16. the energy system that provides the majority of energy in endurance races
18. the watery interior of cells
21. electron carrier molecule known as nicotinamide adenine dinucleotide (abbrev.)

Name: _____   Course Number: _____

Section: _____   Date: _____

CHAPTER 3

Carbohydrates

Daily Carbohydrates and Fiber for Athletes

Use the 1-day meal plan listed below to answer questions in this section.

Breakfast	Carbohydrate (grams)
12 oz orange juice	40
1 large hearty grain bagel	49
2 tbsp peanut butter	7
1 cup oatmeal	27
½ cup soy milk	5
Lunch	
2 cups black bean soup	60
1 piece corn bread	29
2 cups green salad with raw vegetables	25
8 oz tomato juice	12
Snack	
5 halves dried apricots	11
6 oz low-fat yogurt with fruit	30
Dinner	
2 cups macaroni and cheese	80
1 cup steamed carrots	22
12 oz light chocolate soy milk	33
Snack	
1 snack-size bag microwave popcorn	10
12 oz water	0

One-day meal total calories = **2,780**

1. Calculate the percentage of calories from carbohydrates in the entire 1-day meal plan.

2. Compare the calculated percentage to the daily carbohydrate recommendations for athletes. Explain how this meal plan meets or does not meet the established recommendations.

3. Find the items on the 1-day meal plan that contain fiber. Research these food items to determine the total fiber and type of fiber for each item. Place the item and grams of total fiber for each fiber-containing food in the appropriate column below, according to its general fiber classification.

Food Item (total fiber, *insoluble*)	Food Item (total fiber, *soluble*)

4. Determine the total grams of fiber consumed in this 1-day meal plan. Does this amount of fiber meet the recommendations for a healthful diet? Describe why or why not.

5. Describe the health benefits of consuming a high-fiber diet. Include the benefits of both soluble and insoluble fiber.

6. Describe the considerations athletes should make when consuming high-fiber foods while training and competing.

Daily Carbohydrates and Fiber for Athletes

You Are the Nutrition Coach

Please read each case study listed below, and answer the associated questions.

1. Kelly (66 kg) is a 48-year-old race walker who participates in half marathons. She walks 5–6 days per week at a moderate to high intensity. Kelly makes an appointment with you to determine how much carbohydrate she should be consuming daily to keep her glycogen levels as high as possible. She is also interested in knowing how to properly "carbohydrate load" the week before a race.

   Questions: How many grams of carbohydrate would you recommend Kelly consume on a daily basis? What suggestions do you have for Kelly for carbohydrate loading 5–7 days prior to her races?

2. Julie is interested in losing weight. She enjoys participating in step aerobics, kickboxing, and muscle conditioning group fitness classes 4–5 times per week. She eliminated all breads, pastas, and other grains as well as dairy products from her diet 4 months ago to help her lose weight. She lost a couple pounds initially, but has struggled to continue her weight loss. Julie's goal is to lose another 5 pounds while also feeling more energetic during the day at work.

   Questions: Does Julie need to start eating grains and dairy again? Please provide justification for your answer. If she refuses to eat grains and dairy, what would you suggest as an alternative?

3. Justin is a 35-year-old, 165 lb, recreational weight lifter. His goal is to build lean mass and lose fat mass. He is interested in knowing what to consume for recovery after his workouts, since he lifts 5–6 days per week. He is currently drinking a recovery shake that contains 45 grams of protein and 20 grams of carbohydrate.

   Questions: How much carbohydrate does Justin need after his workouts for optimal recovery? Should he continue drinking his recovery shake?

Crossword Puzzle

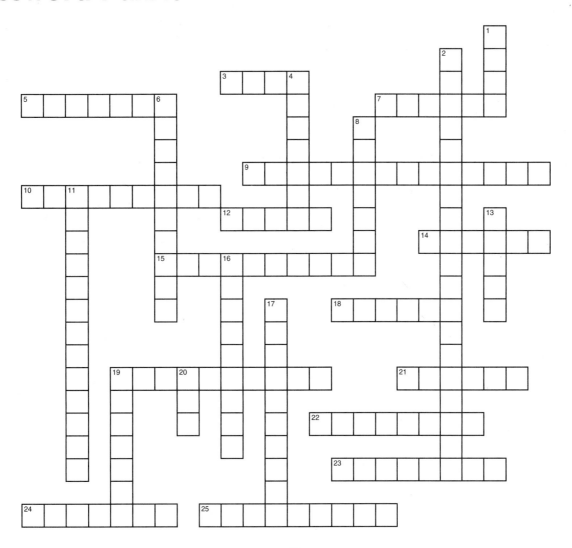

Across

3. generally recognized as safe (abbrev.)
5. this type of fiber has been reported to decrease blood cholesterol levels
7. the storage form of carbohydrates in plants
9. requiring process that forms carbohydrates
10. a commonly used artificial sweetener
12. carbon dioxide is combined with this to form carbohydrates
14. excellent source of fructose
15. low levels of muscle glycogen can result in the early onset of this
18. glucose is this type of sugar
19. formed during the anaerobic breakdown of carbohydrates (2 words)
21. carbohydrates are made in nature by these
22. this index can be used to determine the blood glucose response to a single food
23. the storage form of glucose in humans
24. commonly consumed food that is an excellent source of soluble fiber and carbohydrate
25. the point at which the body starts using more carbohydrates than fats

Down

1. it is best to ingest this type of glycemic index food post-exercise
2. nutritional practice that packs muscle cells with glycogen (2 words)
4. more commonly known as table sugar
6. when coming up with a pre-game or competition meal plan, it is suggested that athletes do this with different foods before the event
8. hormone responsible for increasing glucose uptake by cells
11. the majority of one's total calories should come from these
13. this form of carbohydrate helps move foods through the GI tract
16. a fat cell
17. metabolic pathway that breaks down glucose into pyruvate
19. sugar found in milk
20. glycogen restoration is quicker if carbohydrates are ingested within how many hours post-exercise/competition

Name: _____ Course Number: _____

Section: _____ Date: _____

CHAPTER 4

Fats

The Importance of Fat Intake for Athletes

1. Define the following types of fat. List three food sources of each type of fat.

   a. Monounsaturated

   b. Polyunsaturated

   c. Saturated

   d. Trans fats

2. Which of the four types of fat in the previous question are considered least healthful? Which are considered most healthful? Provide an explanation of your answers.

3. Consider an athlete who for the last month has cut virtually all of the fat out of her diet. She states that her reason for this reduction is because her previously high fat intake was "slowing her down" on the track. Now she consumes mostly fat-free foods, and her daily intake of fat averages 15–20 grams. Is this level of fat intake acceptable? Describe the benefits of consuming adequate fat in an athlete's diet. What changes in dietary intake would you recommend to this athlete?

© 2010 Jones and Bartlett Publishers

You Are the Nutrition Coach

Please read each case study listed below, and answer the associated questions.

1. Calvin is a 19-year-old collegiate gymnast. He has been consuming approximately 3,200 calories per day, feels energetic, recovers well, and has maintained his weight at 150 pounds for the last 2 years. After a recent blood test, he discovered that his total cholesterol is 235. He is concerned about this result, and asks for your assistance in making the necessary dietary changes to lower his cholesterol.

   Questions: How many grams of total fat, as well as saturated, monounsaturated, and polyunsaturated fats, would you recommend Calvin consume daily? Do you have any other dietary suggestions that would help Calvin lower his cholesterol?

2. Therese is a 45-year-old lawyer and masters swimmer. Swim practices are held at 11:30 AM or 6:00 PM at a pool near her office. Therese is frustrated because she gets very hungry during the day, and therefore, has a difficult time swimming strongly throughout either a noon or evening practice. She often leaves practice early because she becomes extremely hungry and sometimes lightheaded. She eats a bagel with fat-free cream cheese and a banana for breakfast, and a turkey sandwich with fat-free yogurt and baby carrots for lunch, every day.

   Questions: Why is Therese so hungry throughout the day? What dietary changes would you recommend to Therese, based on the brief food recall provided? Please include specific meal planning ideas in your answer.

3. Bruce is a road cyclist. He joins his cycling buddies for 80–100 mile rides on the weekends. To stay energized and well-hydrated, he will typically consume water, sports beverages, gels, peanut butter sandwiches, sesame sticks, and trail mix during his long rides. Lately, he has been experiencing some intestinal cramping and diarrhea near the end of his rides, and for several hours after his rides. He is concerned that the simple sugars in the sports beverages and the gels are causing his problems. He asks to meet with you to discuss other sports nutrition products on the market that may help to prevent his gastrointestinal issues.

   Questions: What is your assessment of Bruce's situation? What dietary recommendations would you provide to Bruce for during his long weekend rides?

Crossword Puzzle

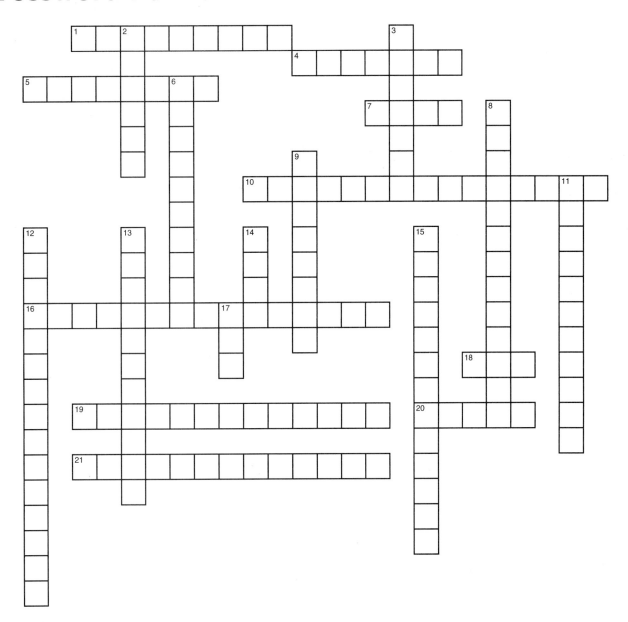

Across

1. type of fatty acid with a full complement of hydrogens attached to its carbons
4. a popular fat substitute composed of sucrose and fatty acids
5. the name of fat surrounding internal organs
7. when a fatty acid is cleaved off of a triglyceride, it becomes this
10. type of fat with two or more double bonds in its carbon chain
16. a blood vessel disease resulting from fatty plaque formation
18. isomeric configuration of most naturally occurring unsaturated fats
19. lipids that are found in the cell membranes of plant and animal tissues
20. type of unsaturated fat associated with increased risk for cardiovascular disease
21. the most common lipids found in the body

Down

2. the minimum percentage of fat recommended in an athlete's total daily calories
3. category of lipids that has hydrocarbon rings in its structure
6. fat cells
8. process that can result in the formation of trans-fats
9. makes up the carbon backbone of triglycerides
11. local hormone-like substances produced from omega 3 fatty acids
12. triglyceride synonym
13. term used to describe the water insolubility of fats
14. the number of calories in 1 gram of fat
15. the body's shift to burning more fats due to a high-fat diet (2 words)
17. a bad cholesterol (abbrev.)

CHAPTER 5

Proteins

Protein Intake for Athletes

Protein Product Comparison

Use the abbreviated label and cost information from skim milk and a protein supplement below to complete this section.

Skim Milk	Whey Protein Supplement
Serving size: 8 ounces	Serving size: 2 scoops
Calories: 90	Calories: 110
Carbohydrate: 12 grams	Carbohydrate: 4 grams
Protein: 8 grams	Protein: 22 grams
Fat: 0 grams	Fat: 0 grams
Vitamin A: 500 IU	Vitamin A: 0 IU
Vitamin D: 100 IU	Vitamin D: 0 IU
Calcium: 300 mg	Calcium: 100 mg
Potassium: 380 mg	Potassium: 170 mg
Cost: $3.90 per gallon	Cost: $36.00 per container (80 scoops)

1. Calculate the cost *per serving* for each product.

2. Which of the two products is the better value based on cost per gram of protein?

3. Compare the nutrient information listed for each product. Which product has a better nutritional value? Explain your answer.

Calculating Protein Recommendations

A 210-pound male basketball player has a goal of losing fat while simultaneously gaining muscle mass and strength.

1. How much protein should this athlete consume daily to meet these goals?

2. List specific recommendations for this athlete regarding types of foods and/or supplements to consume to achieve the daily protein recommendation calculated in (1).

You Are the Nutrition Coach

Please read each case study listed below, and answer the associated questions.

1. Kara is a 14-year-old, 125 lb high school basketball player. She has been feeling fatigued and sore lately, and has been sick three separate times in the last 3–4 months. Kara typically eats the following on a daily basis:

    7 AM: 10–12 oz orange juice (at home before school)

    11:30 AM: 2 cups macaroni and cheese, and a small fruit cup (lunch in school cafeteria)

    3 PM: granola bar (before basketball practice)

    7 PM: 2–3 cups spaghetti with tomato sauce, 1 piece garlic bread, 10 oz skim milk (at home after practice)

    10 PM: 2 cups ice cream (bedtime snack)

    Questions: Why is Kara feeling fatigued, sore and sick? What dietary recommendations would you give to Kara? Please be specific with your recommendation, especially regarding protein intake.

2. Kyle is a collegiate hockey player. He currently weighs 165 lbs, and his goal is to gain 5–10 lbs within the next 2–3 months. In addition to a full class schedule, he practices with the hockey team daily, travels to games on the weekends, and works part-time in the campus bookstore. He wants to know how much protein he should consume daily. Kyle is also interested in meal and snack ideas for his travel weekends with the team.

    Questions: How many grams of protein should Kyle consume daily? Explain your answer. Please provide at least five protein-rich and well-balanced meal/snack ideas for Kyle's travel weekends.

3. Linda is a half marathon runner. She read an article in a runner's magazine promoting a new sports beverage that contains protein. She has always used a traditional carbohydrate-rich sports beverage, and has had great results. However, she wonders if this new product would work even better and help her run faster.

Questions: Would this new sports beverage containing protein work well for Linda? How much protein should Linda be consuming before and during a half marathon?

Crossword Puzzle

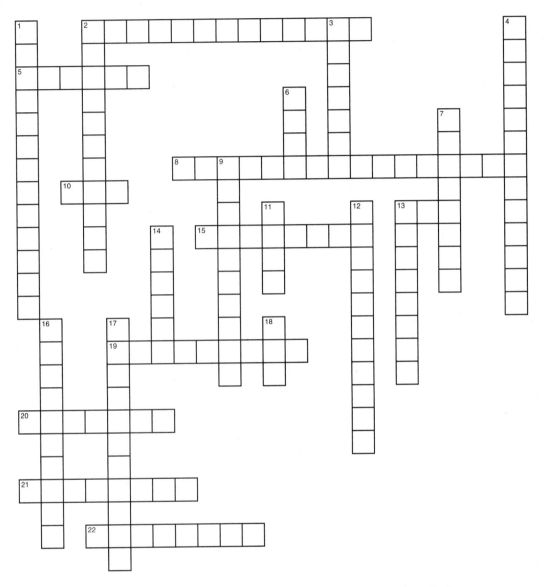

Across

2. adequate intake of these spares dietary protein and muscle tissue
5. number of amino acids used by the human body
8. the sequence of amino acids gives rise to this (2 words)
10. a non-dairy milk that is an excellent source of protein
13. highest recommended daily intake of protein in g/kg of body weight
15. nitrogen status when protein in exceeds protein out
19. amino acids that cannot be synthesized in the body
20. bond that holds amino acids together
21. an essential amino acid that is in short supply is called this
22. high-quality proteins also are this

Down

1. outside of the cell
2. amino acids that become essential but are not normally so
3. dietary proteins are used to make these
4. these amino acids can be metabolized for energy in the muscle (2 words)
6. average caloric value of one gram of protein
7. unlike fats and carbohydrates, proteins contain this
9. another name for a low-quality protein
11. this food group does not contain proteins
12. a high-protein diet can cause this condition
13. this level of protein structure determines the three dimensional shape of a single polypeptide chain
14. makes up the "second string" of dietary sources of protein
16. a three amino acid protein
17. the metabolic process of cleaving off the amino group from an amino acid
18. excessive protein supplementation can increase this component of the body

Name: _____   Course Number: _____

Section: _____   Date: _____

CHAPTER 6

Vitamins

Importance of Vitamin Intake for Athletes

The table below will help you identify the major roles of each vitamin for athletic performance and overall health. Please complete the five categories for each vitamin. An example
is provided for thiamin to guide you in completing this table.

Vitamin: Adult RDA or AI (Male and Female)	Food Sources	Sport Performance Significance	Increased Need in Athletes?	Comments
Thiamin RDA: 1.2 mg M 1.1 mg F	Whole grains, legumes, nuts, pork	Coenzyme—thiamin pyrophosphate converts pyruvate to acetyl CoA	Yes, with increased calorie needs	Needs are based on calorie intake—if athletes are eating enough food to meet their calorie needs, then they are typically consuming adequate amounts of thiamin
Riboflavin				
Niacin				
Vitamin B_{12}				
Vitamin C				
Vitamin A				
Vitamin D				
Vitamin E				
Vitamin K				
Antioxidants				
Vitamins A, C, E	See A, C, and E food sources			

You Are the Nutrition Coach

Please read each case study listed below, and answer the associated questions.

1. Doug is a 56-year-old tri-athlete. A recent physical revealed that his blood levels of homocysteine were elevated. His doctor suggested improving his diet to lower his homocysteine levels. Doug schedules an appointment with you to learn more about the dietary changes required to lower his blood levels of homocysteine.

   Questions: Adequate consumption of which vitamins may help Doug decrease his homocysteine levels? Name three foods or beverages that are rich sources of these vitamins.

2. Sally is a 68-year-old woman who walks 3 times per week, and attends yoga class 2 times per week. She has read several nutrition articles which suggested that women older than 50 years of age take supplemental vitamin D, vitamin B_{12}, choline, and thiamin. Sally asks for your advice in choosing the appropriate supplements.

   Questions: Do you agree with the recommendations from the nutrition articles? If yes, please provide your suggestions for food sources and supplements of vitamin D, vitamin B_{12}, choline, and thiamin. If you do not agree with the nutrition articles, please provide appropriate recommendations for Sally regarding vitamin intake.

3. Tony is a 17-year-old basketball player. His coach recommended that Tony find a supplement to aid in his recovery from workouts. Tony found a product that contains 10 grams of protein, 40 grams of carbohydrate, 1,000 mg of vitamin C, and 30 milligrams of vitamin E per serving.

   Questions: Did Tony find an appropriate supplement to aid in his post-workout recovery? If yes, how many servings should Tony consume after a workout? If not, what recommendations would you provide to Tony for an alternative supplement or food product?

Crossword Puzzle

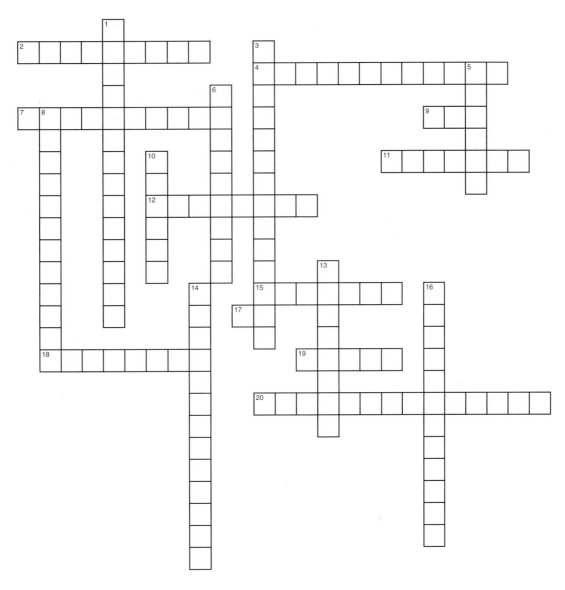

Across

2. fatty acid transporter within cells
4. vitamin B dependent enzymes break down this heart-risky compound
7. these vitamins should not be taken in excess because of toxicity risk (2 words)
9. Recommended Dietary Allowance (abbrev.)
11. this tends to destroy water-soluble vitamins; thus, raw is best
12. tomatoes and pizza sauce contain this carotenoid important for prostate health
15. this energy system is responsible for forming "reactive oxidative species"
17. tolerable upper intake level (abbrev.)
18. vitamin D is sometimes called this vitamin
19. vitamins B and C dissolve in this
20. bumpy, scaly skin caused by a lack of vitamin A

Down

1. vitamins make up part of this category of nutrients
3. potent plant derived antioxidants
5. this B vitamin causes itchy rashes when taken in excess
6. class of compounds important for vision
8. these protect the body from free radicals
10. "foliage" foods are abundant in this vitamin
13. vitamin C is important for the formation of this fibrous protein
14. high calcium levels in the blood
16. highly reactive molecules thought to have negative health effects (2 words)

Name: _____   Course Number: _____

Section: _____   Date: _____

CHAPTER 7

Minerals

Importance of Mineral Intake for Athletes

The table below will help you identify the major roles of minerals for athletic performance and overall health. Please complete the five categories for each mineral. An example is provided for calcium to guide you in completing this table.

Mineral: Adult RDA or AI (Male and Female)	Food Sources	Sport Performance Significance	Increased Need in Athletes?	Comments
Calcium AI: 1,000 mg M 1,000 mg F 19–50 years	Dairy, fortified foods (soy milk, tofu, orange juice), fish with bones	Bone density; prevention of fractures	Not necessarily for athletes; supplementation for athletes only if they are not consuming enough (same protocol as for sedentary individuals). It is fairly common for athletes to not consume enough calcium daily.	For athletes who have been diagnosed with the Female Athlete Triad or osteoporosis, adequate calcium intake or supplementation needed. With supplementation, the body can only absorb ~500 mg dose at one time.
Phosphorus				
Magnesium				
Sodium				
Potassium				
Iron				
Zinc				

Name: _____   Course Number: _____

Section: _____   Date: _____

You Are the Nutrition Coach

Please read each case study listed below, and answer the associated questions.

1. Keri is a 16-year-old cross-country runner who has been referred to you by her physician. Keri has recently lost 20 pounds, is currently amenorrheic, and has been diagnosed with osteopenia.

   Questions: Although all essential minerals are important, which are of particular concern for Keri at this time? Please provide suggestions for specific foods or beverages for Keri to consume daily.

2. Heidi is a 21-year-old collegiate rower. She makes an appointment with you because she has been low in energy lately, and wants to know if her diet may be the reason she is so fatigued. Heidi mentions that she was not allowed to give blood at the campus blood drive because the staff told her that her "iron was too low." She wants to know what that means, and if she should start taking iron supplements.

   Questions: As Heidi's dietitian, what steps would you take to assess her iron status and subsequent nutritional needs? Would you recommend that Heidi begin taking iron supplements?

3. Jay is a 28-year-old accountant and recreational soccer player. He was referred to you by his physician because he has developed a goiter. In your initial phone conversation with Jay, he admits that his busy schedule has led him to eat solely fast food and canned or prepackaged products. He eats very few fruits and vegetables, does not have a sweet tooth, but does love salt and adds it to all his meals. He is frustrated by this recent diagnosis, and is unsure how changing his diet will help improve his condition.

   Questions: Is it possible that Jay's goiter was caused by his diet? If yes, an excess or deficiency of which mineral could have been the culprit? What suggestions would you give to Jay to improve his condition?

Crossword Puzzle

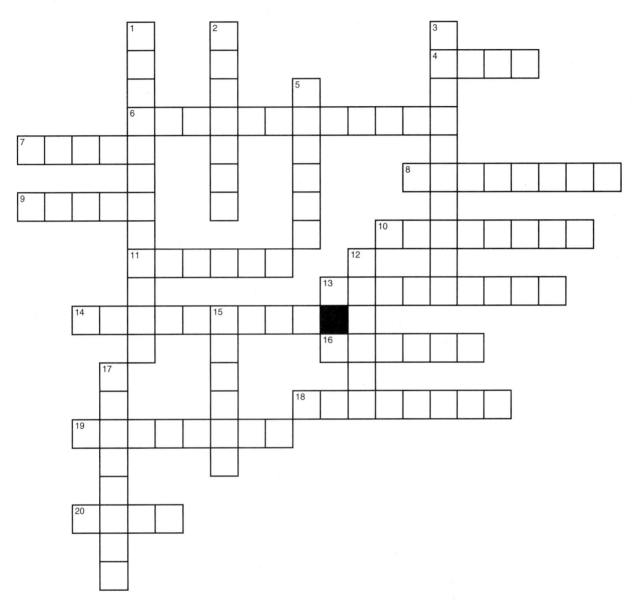

Across

4. type of iron found in meats and animal foods
6. ions that are important to the generation of electrical activity in the body
7. these minerals are needed in amounts greater than 100 mg
8. component part of salt
9. minerals needed by the body in very small quantities
10. enhances the action of insulin
11. one of the most abundant minerals found in sweat
13. bananas are rich in this mineral
14. these substances do not contain carbon in their structure
16. essential mineral with no established DRIs
18. this micronutrient will improve the absorption of non-heme iron
19. excessive intake of this mineral can cause mottling of the teeth
20. important to the function of over 200 enzymes throughout the body

Down

1. excessive intake of sodium can cause this
2. adequate intake of this mineral is critical for bone health
3. mineral important for bone rigidity
5. fortified in salt to help prevent goiter
12. good source of calcium
15. iron deficiency can cause this
17. seafood is high in this mineral, which is considered an antioxidant

CHAPTER 8

Water

Importance of Water Intake for Athletes

Match each word or number with the correct statement regarding fluid needs for athletes. Some terms may be used more than once; others may not be correct for any statement. Each statement may have more than one correct answer.

2	17–20	heat stroke
2.2	250–400 ml	juice
3	500–1,000 ml	milk
5	600–750 ml	sports beverages
7–10	energy drinks	water
16–24	heat exhaustion	water intoxication

1. Amount of water typically obtained from daily food intake. _____

2. Adequate intake of total water for men, older than 19 years (in liters). _____

3. Adequate intake of total water for women, older than 19 years (in liters). _____

4. Urine rating number when urine is a light yellow color. _____

5. Amount of water output typically lost daily from the lungs. _____

6. The amount of fluid, in ounces, that should be consumed 4 hours prior to exercise. _____

7. Excellent fluid choice before exercise. _____

8. Average amount of fluid, in ounces, athletes require every 10–20 minutes during exercise. _____

9. Heat-related disorder that results in a rapid pulse and hypotension. _____

10. Lack of sweat, dry/hot skin, and muscle incoordination are signs and symptoms of this heat-related disorder. _____

11. Percentage of body weight lost when an athlete feels thirsty, uncomfortable, and has a lack of appetite. _____

12. Appropriate fluid choice during exercise. _____

13. Fluid that may be helpful for muscle recovery and rehydration. _____

14. Amount of fluid, in ounces, that should be consumed for every pound of body weight lost during exercise. _____

Determine Your Fluid Needs During Exercise

Record your sweat trial data for 2 exercise sessions; each session should be 30–60 minutes in duration. Choose 2 different modes of exercise; for example, running and weight lifting. Fill in the blanks below to complete your calculations. Evaluate your current fluid intake as compared to your needs, and develop specific goals for improving your hydration during exercise.

Exercise Session #1

1. Determine body weight lost during exercise.

   Body weight before exercise − body weight after exercise = pounds of water weight lost

   _____ − _____ = _____

2. Determine the fluid equivalent, in ounces, of the total weight lost during exercise.

   Pounds of water weight lost during exercise × 16–24 oz = number of ounces of additional fluid that should have been consumed to maintain fluid balance during the exercise session

   _____ × 16–24 oz = _____

3. Determine your actual fluid needs during the workout.

   Ounces of fluid consumed + ounces of additional fluid needed to establish fluid balance = total fluid needs

   _____ + _____ = _____

4. Determine the number of fluid ounces needed per hour of exercise.

   Total fluid needs ÷ total workout time in hours = fluid ounces per hour of exercise

   _____ ÷ _____ = _____

5. Evaluate your current fluid intake as compared to your needs, and develop specific goals for improving your hydration during this type of exercise.

Exercise Session #2

1. Determine body weight lost during exercise.

   Body weight before exercise − body weight after exercise = pounds of water weight lost

   _____ − _____ = _____

2. Determine the fluid equivalent, in ounces, of the total weight lost during exercise.

Pounds of water weight lost during exercise × 16–24 oz = number of ounces of additional fluid that should have been consumed to maintain fluid balance during the exercise session

_____ × 16–24 oz = _____

3. Determine your actual fluid needs during the workout.

Ounces of fluid consumed + ounces of additional fluid needed to establish fluid balance = total fluid needs

_____ + _____ = _____

4. Determine the number of fluid ounces needed per hour of exercise.

Total fluid needs ÷ total workout time in hours = fluid ounces per hour of exercise

_____ ÷ _____ = _____

5. Evaluate your current fluid intake as compared to your needs, and develop specific goals for improving your hydration during this type of exercise.

You Are the Nutrition Coach

Please read each case study listed below, and answer the associated questions.

1. You and your friends are going on a long hike in sunny Moab, Utah, in late May. The hike is the first in a series of endurance training sessions you will do to prepare for the Pikes Peak Ascent (a half marathon to the top of Pikes Peak, 14,000 ft) in Colorado Springs in mid-August. The average daytime temperature in Moab in May is 85°F, and the relative humidity averages 20%. You plan to be gone on the hike for 3 hours. You have a pack that is large enough to carry sufficient fluids for your personal needs for the duration of the hike.

   Questions:

   a. How will the environmental conditions in Moab affect your fluid needs during this training hike?

   b. What fluid recommendations should you and your friends follow before, during, and after this 3-hour training hike? Your recommendations should begin 2 hours prior to the hike, and continue through 1-hour post-hike. In your answer, include the guidelines for both the amount and type of fluid needed.

2. Tina lives in central Illinois, and has competed in several triathlons each summer for the last 4 years. Her times have improved greatly, and she often places in the top 5 women in shorter, local races. She has decided to try longer distance triathlons this year with the goal of competing in the August Half Ironman Triathlon in Nashville, Tennessee. It is now early March, and the Nashville Half Ironman Triathlon is scheduled for late August. She tells you she has a hard time hydrating during training because it is too cumbersome to carry fluid with her while running, and when she's on her bike, she often forgets to drink unless she is really thirsty. She asks you to help her develop an appropriate, yet practical, hydration plan.

Questions:

a. You ask Tina to perform a sweat trial during an upcoming 2-hour training session to determine how much fluid she should consume during training. Use the information below to calculate her fluid needs *per hour*.

Height: 5'8"

Weight prior to the workout: 138 lbs

Weight after the 2-hour workout: 135 lbs

Tina consumed 24 oz of fluid during the 2-hour workout; she did not urinate during the workout.

b. What should Tina do to ensure proper hydration during high mileage, outdoor workouts during the hot and humid summer months leading up to the triathlon in August?

c. What signs or symptoms should Tina be aware of that may indicate she is not adequately hydrated daily or during workouts?

Crossword Puzzle

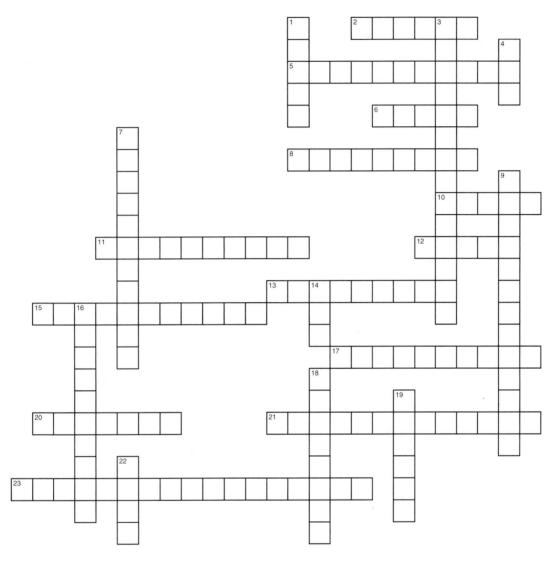

Across

2. low blood levels of this can lead to hyponatremia
5. results from a negative water balance
6. important to evaporative cooling
8. water can be lost particularly at high altitudes during this process
10. formation of this is a major avenue of water loss at rest
11. severe condition in which the body stops sweating and body temperature soars out of control (2 words)
12. 55–60% of body weight is this
13. type of water formed during the aerobic breakdown of macronutrients
15. performing these under different environmental conditions will help establish a hydration plan for athlete (2 words)
17. water lost via seepage through the skin is said to be this
20. this type of "drift" occur as the athlete becomes dehydrated and loses blood volume
21. lymph and blood plasma are this type of water
23. hyponatremia (2 words)

Down

1. drinks that should be avoided prior to exercise
3. group of athletes at risk for hyponatremia
4. recommended water intake in milliliters per calorie of energy expended
7. a negative water balance increases the risk for these disorders (2 words)
9. water found inside cells
14. number of cups of water needed to offset a 1-lb weight loss due to sweating
16. an athlete in "fluid balance" is said to be this
18. supplementation of these can change urine color and give the impression of a dehydrated state
19. urine that is a dark shade of this would suggest dehydration
22. for some athletes this is an excellent choice for pre-exercise hydration

CHAPTER 9

Nutritional Ergogenics

Nutritional Ergogenics for Athletic Performance

1. Go online and search for a *nutritional* supplement (not a drug) that is targeted toward athletes. Choose any supplement that appears interesting and promotes some physiological benefit to athletic performance. Critique the advertisement and the product using the guidelines below. Turn in a copy of the advertisement with your critique.

Nutritional Supplement Critique Guidelines:

- List the supplement's name, category of supplement, and price per serving.

- Describe the claimed actions for athletic performance.

- Critique the claimed actions:
  - Analyze the claimed benefits using what you know about physiology and biochemistry. Is there research from scientifically sound sources to support the product's claims? Describe the quality of the research on the supplement and/or ingredients.

- Is the advertisement based on testimonials only?

- Determine safety issues of the supplement and/or ingredients contained in the supplement. Is the supplement or its ingredients banned by any sports or athletic organizations?

- Determine if you would recommend this supplement to an athlete, and describe why or why not.

2. Which athletes are most likely to benefit from taking a multivitamin/mineral supplement?

© 2010 Jones and Bartlett Publishers

You Are the Nutrition Coach

Please read each case study listed below, and answer the associated questions.

1. Louise is a 42-year-old woman who enjoys Pilates, yoga, tennis, and strength training with her personal trainer. For several years, she has been taking the following supplements:

   - Daily multivitamin/mineral

   - 500 mg potassium

   - B-complex vitamin

   - 50 μg chromium

   - 400 mg magnesium

   - 500 mg calcium, twice per day

   - 200 IU vitamin D, twice per day

   - 25 mg zinc

   These supplements have been recommended to her from a variety of sources, including friends, family, past personal trainers, and the woman from whom she purchases her supplements. Louise is interested in knowing how she is doing with her diet, and if she needs any additional supplements considering her age and level of activity.

   Questions: Please evaluate the profile of supplements Louise is currently taking on a daily basis. Which supplements would you recommend that she continue to take and which products should she discontinue using?

2. Dustin is a 22-year-old race car driver. In preparation for the racing season, Dustin would like to lose 5–10 lbs. He is mainly interested in losing body fat. At a local health food store, a sales representative suggested that he try a supplement with yohimbe. Dustin asks if you would also recommend yohimbe as a natural way to help him meet his goals.

   Questions: Would you recommend that Dustin take the product containing yohimbe? Why or why not? Would you recommend any other supplements to Dustin to help him reach his goals?

3. Bob is 37 years old, and has just joined the fire department. Since his new job requires him to be strong and powerful, he has started a new strength training routine. He has heard from other firefighters, as well as guys at the gym, that he should be taking a protein supplement to maximize his results from working out so hard in the weight room. He has researched some products online that contain whey, casein, soy, glutamine, and leucine. He makes an appointment with you to discuss which product will be best in helping him to recover from workouts and build muscle mass.

Questions: What are your recommendations for Dustin? Provide Dustin with several reputable online sources that may help him to research supplements in the future.

Crossword Puzzle

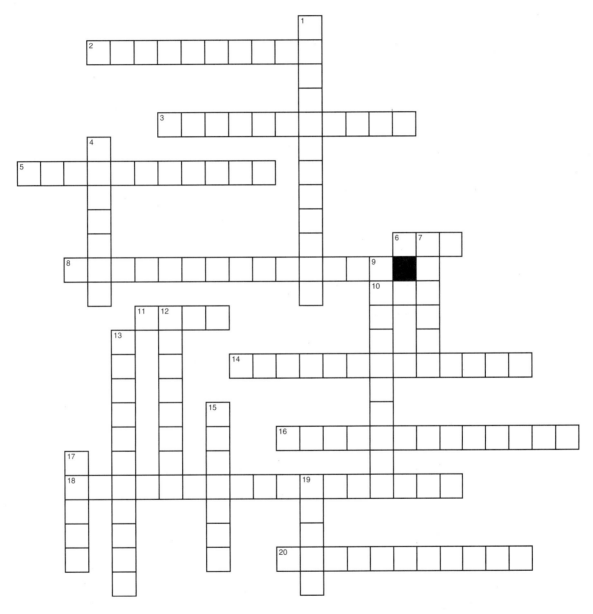

Across

2. a hormone precursor
3. reference database dedicated to sports medicine and other exercise related areas
5. adage that should apply to all dietary supplements (2 words)
6. if a manufacturer makes a health claim, then the product must be approved by this agency (abbrev.)
8. these compounds slow down the body's breakdown processes
10. agency that verifies quality manufacturing practices (abbrev.)
11. international agency that seeks to control doping practices (abbrev.)
14. strength training is an example of this type of ergogenic aid
16. oversized golf club heads represent this type of ergogenic aid
18. these claims do not need any governmental approval (2 words)
20. the FTC regulates this area of the supplement industry

Down

1. commonly used by supplement manufacturers to sell product
4. the premier database of the U.S. National Library of Medicine
7. the act of using foreign substances to improve performance
9. a dietary product that is not intended to be used as a food
12. these substances cause increases in protein synthesis and muscle mass
13. doping that occurs when an athlete unknowingly takes a supplement that contains a banned substance
15. a source of ephedrine (2 words)
17. legislation regulating the supplement industry (abbrev.)
19. United States equivalent to the World Anti-Doping Agency (abbrev.)

CHAPTER 10

Nutrition Consultation with Athletes

Consulting with Athletes

1. Describe the advantages and disadvantages of having athletes complete a 1-, 3-, and 7-day food record. List and briefly describe at least 2 other methods of collecting dietary intake information from athletes to aid in conducting nutrition consultations.

2. The 1-day food record below is from a male athlete who is trying to "eat better to be able to work out harder during soccer practice." You have reviewed the 1-day record and have started your first consultation with him. What information do you need to clarify with the athlete about his diet? List 5 specific questions you will ask him, and describe why you would ask each question.

1-Day Food Record

Breakfast

1 bagel with cream cheese

1 cup orange juice

1 bowl dry cereal

1 cup milk

Lunch

2 ham and cheese sandwiches

1 bag potato chips

1 large apple

3 chocolate chip cookies

Dinner

2 cups macaroni and cheese

3 spears cooked broccoli

1 roll with butter

1 diet soda

1. _____

2. _____

3. _____

4. _____

5. _____

3. Briefly describe each of the seven steps of the initial nutrition consultation interview process. In your description, list each step, give a brief summary of each step, and the primary reason each step is used in the consultation process.

1. _____

2. _____

3. _____

4. _____

5. _____

6. _____

7. _____

4. You are a summer intern for a large, reputable sports beverage company. The company is the primary sponsor of an Olympic-distance triathlon in August in Iowa. The company will have a huge exhibit booth at the prerace meal the night before the race, and before, during, and after the event on race day. Your responsibility as an intern is to create a sports nutrition table display to be the centerpiece of the company's main exhibit area. Describe in detail what the table set-up will look like, the information and activities you will have available for participants, and the main emphasis of your educational message for this athlete population.

Name: _____   Course Number: _____

Section: _____   Date: _____

You Are the Nutrition Coach

Please read each case study listed below, and answer the associated questions.

1. A potential client named Tom calls your office on a Monday morning. He has been looking for a sports dietitian, and he found information on your Web site related to individual nutrition counseling. He states that he is a competitive athlete, and is interested in ensuring that he is consuming enough food to perform well and stay healthy.

   Question: What questions would you ask Tom to learn more about him before scheduling the initial consultation?

2. Marie is a 42-year-old race walker. She contacts you inquiring about private consultations for weight management and athletic performance. She travels around the country to compete in 10K and half marathon road races. Her goals include losing 15 lbs, preventing muscle cramps during long walks, and improving her recovery from weight training workouts. She is interested in scheduling monthly meetings with you to ensure her own accountability.

   Question: What topics will you cover in your monthly consultations with Marie? Create a suggested schedule of topics for her first six sessions.

Crossword Puzzle

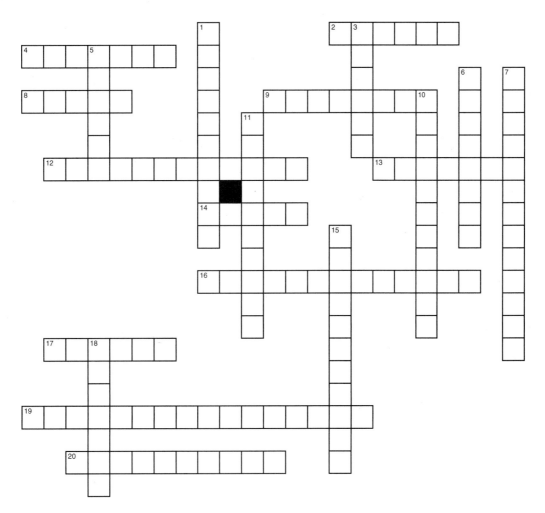

Across

2. these types of nutritional consultation sessions are usually brief and more educational in nature
4. resolving to cut out midnight snacking is an example of this type of oriented goal
8. this legislative act protects the security and privacy of health-related data (abbrev.)
9. when having athletes record their food intake, it is important that the size of these be recorded
12. besides food intake data, the dietitian also should look at these to help in developing the nutritional plan (2 words)
13. when consulting with an athlete, it is important to break down any barriers and establish this with the athlete
14. recommended number of days suggested to adequately assess dietary intake
16. a food intake questionnaire that determines how often common foods are eaten (2 words)
17. this method of dietary data collection requires a person to remember what they ate 24 hours before the consultation
19. transtheoretical stage in which the athlete has no intention of making a change
20. the "R" in RD stands for this

Down

1. these are frequently omitted when food records are being recorded by athletes
3. stage of change in which the athlete is overtly working to modify their diet
5. in order for a nutritional plan to work, it is important to establish whether the athlete is ready for this
6. it is critical to the success of achieving goals that the athletes be allowed to schedule this with the dietitian
7. information about current and past medical issues are usually collected using this type of questionnaire (2 words)
10. it is important to determine whether athletes are taking these when performing a dietary analysis
11. the most commonly used method of collecting nutritional intake data (2 words)
15. a comprehensive form of dietary intake data collection requiring a trained interviewer (2 words)
18. these individuals serve as a common source of nutrition information for athletes

CHAPTER 11

Weight Management

Weight Management for Athletes

1. Fill in the table below. Measure your height, weight, and waist circumference, and place the measurements in the appropriate place on the table.

Your Measurements	Your Body Mass Index	Your BMI Classification
Height: _____		
Weight: _____		
	Ideal waist circumference for women	**Ideal waist circumference for men**
Waist circumference: _____		

Using the information you entered in the table, explain how your measurements compare to BMI and waist circumference standards. What do the standards for both BMI and waist circumference measures mean in relation to health?

2. If a football defensive tackle has a BMI of 31.5, would he need to lose weight? Justify your answer.

3. Place the correct body composition measurement method into the blanks below.

_____ Based on determination of body density; measures body volume by applying Archimedes' Principle.

_____ Uses a three-component model measuring fat mass, bone mineral mass, and lean body mass by passing low-energy radiography technology.

_____ Measures subcutaneous fat at several anatomical sites. A prediction equation is then applied to determine overall body fat percentage.

_____ Determines body volume by air displacement, and uses the volume measure and body weight measure to determine overall body density.

_____ A small electrical current is passed through the body, and a measurement of the resistance to flow of the current is taken.

4. Calculate the pounds of fat mass (FM) and fat-free mass (FFM) using the following information from a male athlete:

Weight: 185 lbs

Body fat: 12%

If this athlete wants to reduce his body fat to 9%, how much weight would he need to lose?

5. Describe the main guidelines athletes should follow to lose weight without decreasing sport performance.

6. Explain each component of the female athlete triad. Include in your explanation of each component: a definition of the component; a brief description of the physical and/or mental health consequences of the component; and the effects on sport performance.

7. Describe the warning signs, medical symptoms, and behaviors that may indicate an athlete (male or female) is struggling with an eating disturbance/disorder.

You Are the Nutrition Coach

Please read each case study listed below, and answer the associated questions.

1. Katrina is a 28-year-old tri-athlete. Her training partner suggested that she make an appointment with you to discuss her nutrition. Katrina complains about being cold all the time, and her friend believes it is because she is too skinny. Katrina claims that she feels full of energy, has no problem getting through training sessions, and is performing quite well in races. She feels good about her nutrition and her current weight, and therefore she does not really see a need to make any changes.

    Questions: With the information you have at this point, what is your initial assessment of the situation? What additional information do you need to collect about Katrina before her first appointment with you?

2. Jerry is a 20-year-old racecar driver. He currently weighs 175 lbs and is 5'7" tall. He would like to lose weight to improve his driving performance and so he can fit into the car more comfortably. He is a full-time student at a local college, and spends his free time at the garage with his racing team. Due to his busy schedule, he eats out for lunch and dinner every day. His goal is to lose 15–20 lbs within the next 4–6 months.

    Questions: Do you support Jerry's goal to lose weight? Please provide three specific suggestions you would give Jerry to help him reach his goal of weight loss.

3. Max is a 16-year-old tennis player. His mother, Linda, calls you to schedule an appointment for Max. He wants to gain 10–20 lbs of weight, but is having a hard time putting on even an ounce. Max is currently 6' tall and weighs 135 lbs. He is in his off-season and, therefore, is not doing any exercise. Linda is frustrated because Max is a very picky eater, which severely limits his food options. While Max has agreed to see a dietitian, he has told his mom that he is most interested in knowing about some quick, easy, weight gain options.

    Questions: What advice and recommendations would you give to Max, based on the information provided in the case study?

Crossword Puzzle

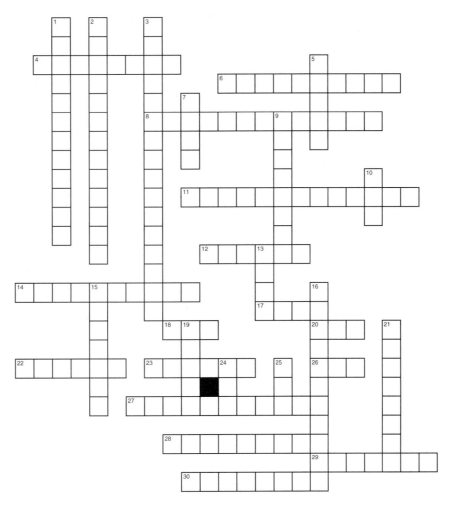

Across

4. high levels of protein intake can do this to fat mass
6. absence of normal menstruation
8. if you are in this, you will neither gain or lose weight (2 words)
11. rapid weight loss in preparation for a competition (2 words)
12. feeling of the need for food derived from physiological cues
14. sport in which eating disorders are prevalent
17. used to measure both bone mineral density and body composition (abbrev.)
18. weekly weight loss, in athletes, should not exceed this number of pounds per week
20. the processes of digestion and absorption of food cause this (abbrev.)
22. air displacement is measured with this
23. body mass index threshold for obesity
26. the largest portion of the total daily energy expenditure (abbrev.)
27. regardless of the dietary composition, controlling this has a big impact on calorie consumption (2 words)
28. carries the name "anorexia" but does not meet actual clinical criteria to be classified as an eating disorder
29. feeling of fullness that lingers after a meal
30. skinfold measures are taken with these

Down

1. the fat found in adipose tissues
2. extra calories for gaining weight should come primarily from these
3. bodybuilders are at a higher risk for this condition (2 words)
5. disordered eating plays a role in the female athlete _____
7. treatment for eating disorders in athletes is best accomplished using this approach
9. a psychologically derived drive to eat
10. uses mild electrical current to determine body composition (abbrev.)
13. underwater weighing is considered to be this standard in regard to body composition determination
15. fat distribution pattern in which waist girth is larger than hip girth
16. skeletal muscle makes up a large part of this (3 words)
19. measuring this can give an indication of the risk for cardiovascular and other serious health-related diseases
21. this type of energy balance is required in order to gain weight
24. pounds of fat lost if at a negative energy balance of 7000 calories
25. a rough indicator of body composition (abbrev.)

CHAPTER 12

Endurance and Ultra-Endurance Athletes

Working with Endurance and Ultra-Endurance Athletes

1. Describe the concept of "hitting the wall" or "bonking" as it relates to energy (macronutrient) utilization in exercise. List the macronutrients that are the primary fuel sources during exercise, and describe what occurs to cause fatigue during long duration exercise.

2. Calculate the range of daily calorie needs using the WHO equation and the following information:

   Female ultra-endurance runner

   5'6" tall; 128 lbs; 34 years old

   In high level training (≥ 3–4 hours per day) in preparation for a 100-mile event in 6 weeks

   Based on your calculation's range of calories, select a calorie level that you think fits her calorie needs. Justify why you selected the calorie level.

3. Complete the table below with the correct levels of macronutrients required for a competitive amateur endurance athlete.

	Daily Grams/kg	Daily % of Total Calories	Before Exercise	During Exercise	After Exercise
Carbohydrate					
Protein					
Fat					

You Are the Nutrition Coach

Please read each case study listed below, and answer the associated questions.

1. Casey is a 37-year-old runner. He is training for his first marathon. He has heard from his experienced running partners that he should eat a lot of pasta in the days before the marathon. He wants to know how much pasta he should eat, and if there is anything else he should focus on, nutritionally, in the days leading up to his race.

    Questions: Describe for Casey how carbohydrate loading can benefit endurance athletes' sport performance. What other tips would you give to Casey in preparation for his marathon?

2. Brittany is a 52-year-old tri-athlete. She has been participating in half Ironman-distance triathlons for several years. She is planning on competing in four races this year, and would like to qualify for the national competition in the fall. In hopes of improving her performance, she has made an appointment with you to review her nutrition during workouts and races. She provides you with a sketch of her usual intake (and race times) during a half Ironman:

    Swim (1:40): no food or drink

    Bike (3:00): three 16 oz bottles of water, two high-protein energy bars, and a peanut butter sandwich

    Run (1:50): sips of water at every aid station, 1–2 gels

    Questions: What is your initial assessment of Brittany's nutrition during workouts/races? What can she change to improve her race day nutrition?

3. Patel is an adventure racer and open water swimmer. He is working with a coach, and is training 20–25 hours per week. To improve his health and athletic performance, his coach has recommended the following supplements:

    B-complex vitamin (for energy): once per day, each pill containing 10 mg thiamin, 10 mg riboflavin, 100 mg niacin, 15 mg vitamin B_6, and 40 μg vitamin B_{12}

    Vitamin C (for recovery): 2,000 mg, twice per day

    Potassium (to prevent cramping): 400 mg per day

    Iron (to improve aerobic endurance): 18 mg, twice per day

    Questions: Please evaluate Patel's supplement regimen. What are your recommendations to Patel regarding his supplement usage?

Crossword Puzzle

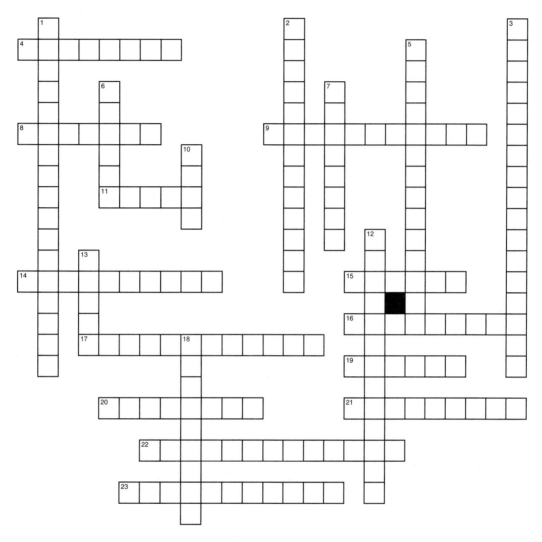

Across

4. the macronutrient content of the extra calories needed by endurance athletes should be this
8. hitting the wall
9. having athletes carry one at all times can help prevent dehydration (2 words)
11. athletes should perform these trials in order to help determine their daily fluid intake
14. dietary practice of purposely ingesting high levels of fat (2 words)
15. most Americans and athletes consume plenty of this electrolyte on a daily basis
16. consumption of these triglycerides is not recommended during exercise (2 words)
17. elite endurance athletes possess this (2 words)
19. an excellent source of potassium
20. a planned decrease in the intensity and volume of training in the days leading up to a competition
21. breakdown of red blood cells
22. these amino acids are theorized to delay onset of fatigue (2 words)
23. how soon after training or competition athletes should begin to ingest carbohydrates

Down

1. this type of endurance represents the ability of the heart and lungs to deliver blood and oxygen to the working muscles
2. this process is required in order to determine individual tolerances and optimal nutrition practices for athletes (3 words)
3. of a muscle or group of muscles to perform without fatigue (2 words)
5. long-distance sport not conducive to eating or drinking (2 words)
6. a great source of carbohydrate during carbohydrate loading
7. these are a good source of sodium and carbohydrates
10. it is very unlikely that the body's stores of these will be depleted during endurance events
12. a relatively cheap recovery drink (2 words)
13. term that describes endurance athletes that participate in events lasting more than four hours
18. as muscle glycogen level decreases, perceived exertion does this

CHAPTER 13

Strength/Power Athletes

Working with Strength/Power Athletes

1. Using information from the previous chapters as well as Chapter 13, list and describe the three main diet/exercise components necessary for an athlete to gain weight.

   1. _____

   2. _____

   3. _____

2. A strength/power athlete who is trying to gain a small amount of weight, primarily as muscle mass, should consume approximately:

   _____   calories per day more than current calorie intake

   _____   grams of carbohydrate per kg body weight

   _____   grams of protein per kg body weight

   _____   percent of total calorie intake as fat

   Provide a justification for your answers to each of the entries above.

3. Devin is an 18-year-old high school track athlete who competes in field events. His specialties are the shot put and discus. He was ranked 12th in the state in shot put as a junior. His goal is to win the state championship this year as a senior. He has 6 months to train before the regional and state meets. He plans to gain 5–8 pounds of muscle mass in the next 2 months so that during peak training, he will be bigger and stronger. However, he has not yet implemented any dietary changes that would initiate the weight gain process. His current intake is listed in the table on page 90. He is 5'11" and weighs 210 lbs. Complete the table below with a revised meal plan that will help Devin meet his weight gain goal. Please document the justification for any changes in the third column.

Sample Meal Plan: Devin

Current: Meals/Snacks	Revised: Meals/Snacks	Reason for Change

Breakfast:
Raisin Bran cereal, 1.5 c
1% milk, 1 c
2 eggs, fried in butter
Orange juice, 12 oz
   Breakfast Total:
   Total Calories: 798
   Protein (g): 31		

Lunch:
Ham sandwiches (3–4 oz), 2
Potato chips, 1 oz pkg
Large apple, 1
Cola, 12 oz
   Lunch Total:
   Total Calories: 953
   Protein (g): 48		

Snack:
Protein shake, ready to drink, 1
(12 oz)
   Snack Total:
   Total Calories: 220
   Protein (g): 22		

Dinner:
Baked fish, 8 oz
Broccoli, cooked, 1 cup
Wild rice, 1 cup
Cola, 12 oz
   Dinner Total:
   Total Calories: 660
   Protein (g): 61		

Snack:
Usually no evening snack
   Snack Total:
   Total Calories: 0
   Protein (g): 0		

Total Daily Intake: Total Calories: 2,631 Protein (g): 162		

You Are the Nutrition Coach

Please read each case study listed below, and answer the associated questions.

1. Alexis is a 14-year-old gymnast. Her days are extremely busy. She wakes up at 7:00 AM and needs to be at school by 7:30 AM. Breakfast is usually eaten in the car on the way to school; lunch is purchased in the school cafeteria. The school day lasts until 3:00 PM, after which she heads to the gym. Practice runs from 3:30 PM until 7:00 PM. After her parents pick her up from the gym, they typically go to a casual dining or fast-food restaurant for dinner. Once Alexis arrives at home, she has 1–2 hours to complete her homework and prepare for the next day. She is frustrated by always eating on the run. Alexis is also concerned that her convenience food diet is not fueling her body properly for gymnastics.

   Questions: Provide two options for quick, healthy meals/snacks for each of the following: breakfast, lunch, afternoon snack, and dinner. Nutrition recommendations should be appropriate for the sport of gymnastics. Suggestions can be given to both Alexis and her parents.

2. Julie is a 51-year-old 800-meter sprinter. She enjoys participating in USA Track & Field events as a masters-level athlete. At the age of 45, Julie suffered a mild stroke. Luckily, she has had to deal with very few long-term complications; the one exception is a slight difficulty with swallowing. While she has been able to regain her strength for training and competing, it has been challenging for her to chew and swallow enough food, in a timely fashion, to fuel her body immediately before events. On race morning, she typically travels to the track, spends plenty of time warming up, and then relaxes before her event. Because of the busy race morning schedule, it has become difficult to have enough time to eat since it takes her longer to chew and swallow. She is looking for ideas for portable, easy-to-consume meals/snacks that she can bring to the track to fuel her running.

   Question: What are your recommendations for Julie? Please provide at least three options for her pre-race meal.

Name: _____ Course Number: _____

Section: _____ Date: _____

Crossword Puzzle

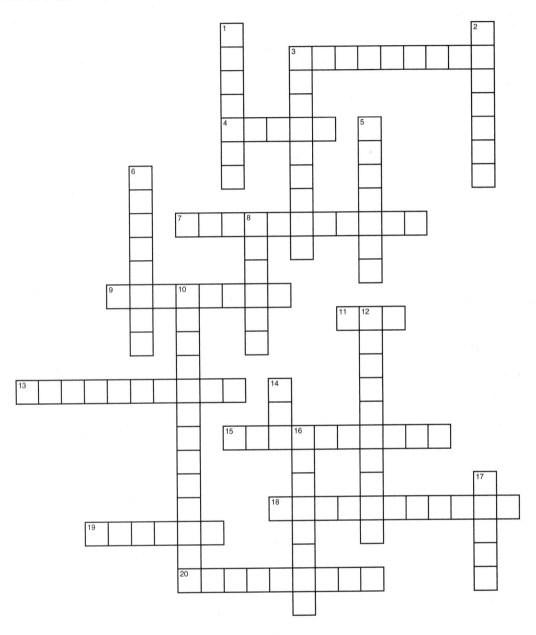

Across

3. blood in the urine
4. mineral that claims to increase testosterone levels
7. after training, when post-exercise feedings should start
9. depleted muscle stores of this can lead to poor strength/power performance
11. excessive protein intake can increase body levels of this
13. dehydration practices cause this (2 words)
15. energy system most important to strength/power athletes
18. excessive protein intake can lead to this condition
19. a hormone released by the pituitary gland in response to resistance training
20. this group of track athletes would epitomize speed/strength

Down

1. energy system responsible for recovery after activity
2. mineral that may aid in fat loss and provides for healthy bones
3. breakdown of red blood cells
5. fats in the diet add to this sense or feeling
6. the type of metabolic process that results in tissue growth
8. train hard and eat well, but neither in _____
10. macronutrient most important to strength/power athletes
12. increased availability of these has been shown to stimulate protein synthesis (2 words)
14. maximum recommended rate of weight gain (pounds per week)
16. a person's maximal bench press would be an indicator of this
17. synonym to speed-strength

CHAPTER 14

Team Sport Athletes

Working with Team Sport Athletes

1. Similar to endurance and strength/power athletes, individuals participating in team sports need to be mindful about their total calorie, macronutrient, and micronutrient intake. Provide a summary of the factors you should consider as you determine the calorie and macronutrient requirements for the various members of an American football team.

2. List at least five ways coaches, trainers, and dietitians can help team members stay well-hydrated during outdoor practices in hot and humid conditions.

3. Planning and preparation are required for team sport athletes who travel to competitive events. You are in charge of arranging the restaurant stops and packing the team coolers for an upcoming trip. The team will be traveling from Evanston, Illinois, to Lincoln, Nebraska, for a weekend tournament. Provide a recommendation for one restaurant stop along the travel route, as well as a restaurant where the team will eat on Saturday evening in Lincoln. Name each restaurant and the reason for your selection.

Make a list of items you would pack in the team cooler. Explain why you are choosing each of these items.

You Are the Nutrition Coach

Please read each case study listed below, and answer the associated questions.

1. Jake is a collegiate soccer player. His team has just completed a very successful season. They are moving into their off-season, during which their workouts are unstructured to allow for rest and recovery. Jake is interested in continuing to stay in shape and to eat healthfully. He has made an appointment with you to determine how he should modify his diet based on his change in workouts.

   Question: Assuming Jake is 20 years old and weighs 165 pounds, calculate his daily calorie, protein, carbohydrate, and fat requirements for the off-season.

2. Erin's softball team has five weekend tournaments that are out-of-state and will require long-distance travel. The team will travel by bus for most of these trips, leaving Friday at noon and returning Sunday around 10:00 PM.

   Question: Provide a brief summary of the foods and/or beverages Erin should bring with her on these trips, and describe why you are suggesting these options.

3. You are conducting a presentation for a local high school football team and their parents. The session is primarily focused on what and how much the players should be consuming before, during, and after their games. After the presentation, you are reviewing the audience's evaluations of the session. One of the parents suggests that next time you include information on how parents can make healthy choices at the concession stands.

   Question: Provide the information you will add to your presentation for next time, to include healthy concession stand choices for the parents of athletes.

Crossword Puzzle

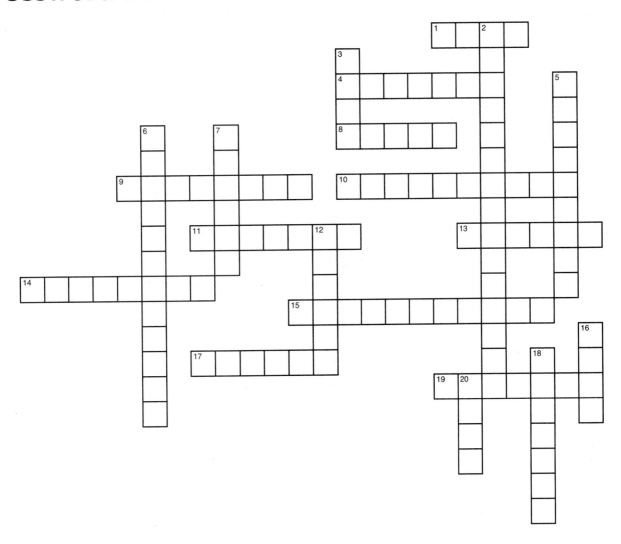

Across

1. category of sport involving multiple athletes playing together against opponents
4. this energy system is important during recovery
8. in some instances, these drinks may be better to consume than plain water
9. ensuring that team athletes stay well-nourished when on the road requires this
10. energy system responsible for supplying ATP during high-intensity activity such as kicking, jumping, or sprinting
11. adequate hydration can be enhanced if coaches/trainers provide a _____ of fluid options
13. these meals are good options for athletes with pre-game jitters
14. doing this every day before and after practice can indicate whether athletes are staying hydrated
15. type of fats recommended for athletes with high-energy needs
17. contrary to the cold environment the sport is played in, these athletes need to make sure they stay well-hydrated
19. diets that meet an athlete's energy needs also will more than likely meet vitamin and ____ needs

Down

2. it takes an athlete's body about 5 days (minimum) for this adjustment to occur
3. these should make up a low caloric percentage of pre-game meals
5. consumption of these types of amino acids after practice have been shown to be beneficial
6. this once-daily "type of" supplement can be taken by team sport athletes as an insurance policy for meeting the RDA
7. ingesting carbohydrates during sport competition has been shown to decrease this type of fatigue
12. at a minimum, during activity athletes should drink every ___ minutes
16. temperature wise, it is better to drink fluids that are this
18. for most team sport athletes, 1.2–1.7 g/kg of this on a daily basis will be acceptable
20. intramuscular triglycerides (abbrev.)

CHAPTER 15

Special Populations

Special Populations Within Athletics

1. Susan is a 15-year-old middle distance track and cross-country runner on her high school team. She was diagnosed with Type 1 diabetes 3 months ago during the off-season. Now the cross-country season has started, and she plans to train and compete just as hard as last year, prior to her diabetes diagnosis.

   Questions:

   a. List the guidelines Susan should follow prior to initiating exercise. Include in your answer glucose and ketone levels, as well as recommendations for exercise dependent upon on those levels.

   b. You are the dietitian or athletic trainer for Susan's cross-country team. You are aware of her recent diabetes diagnosis, and she has shared with you her medications and current dietary regimen. Describe your role in helping Susan optimize her performance by training and competing safely. How do you prepare for the possibility of a diabetic emergency on the track?

2. There are special considerations for children and young teens regarding hydration during exercise in the heat. Why are young athletes potentially at greater risk for dehydration during exercise? What steps can be taken to avoid these concerns?

Name: _____ Course Number: _____

Section: _____ Date: _____

You Are the Nutrition Coach

Please read each case study listed below, and answer the associated questions.

1. Leslie is 45 years old, 5'10", and weighs 140 lbs. She enjoys playing volleyball, soccer, basketball, and racquetball. Four months ago, she partially tore her right gastrocnemius muscle in a basketball game. The doctor told her that the injury would take 4–6 weeks to heal; it has now been 4 months and the injury seems to be worsening. Her doctor recommends that she make an appointment with you to determine if there is a nutritional cause for the lack of healing. You perform a 24-hour recall with Leslie which reveals the following typical day:

    Breakfast: small latte with skim milk and a bagel

    Lunch: large bowl of carrot soup with saltine crackers

    Snack: 1 cup snack mix

    Dinner: Thai take-out (noodle and vegetable dish in a peanut sauce)

    Evening snack: 1 cup low-fat ice cream

    Questions: Based on her 24-hour recall, is she nutritionally deficient in any macronutrient or micronutrient? What dietary changes would you suggest to Leslie that would help to enhance her healing?

2. Henry is a 68-year-old long-distance runner. He enjoys participating in local races nearly every weekend during the spring, summer, and fall. Over the past year, he has struggled with a slight discomfort in his left knee. Henry made an appointment with his doctor to discuss the pain, and was diagnosed with arthritis. Henry is determined to continue with his training and racing plan for the year. He comes to you to find out if there are any foods that he can eat to remedy his arthritis, or at least decrease the pain and stiffness in his knee.

    Questions: What are your recommendations for Henry? Which foods might be beneficial in managing his arthritis?

3. Virginia has been referred to you by her gynecologist. Virginia's doctor is concerned because, not only has she not gained any weight in her first trimester, she has actually lost 4 lbs. Her doctor's second concern is that her recent blood test revealed that she is now anemic. Virginia enjoys swimming three times per week, yoga twice a week, and walking with her girlfriends twice a week. She states that she is feeling great and is having fun being active. Virginia claims that she has been eating more lately; she has added a midafternoon snack of fresh fruit, and a glass of milk before bed. You ask her to record a 3-day food log and email it to you as soon as possible.

Questions: Which macronutrients and micronutrients should you focus on when analyzing her 3-day food log? Has Virginia added enough food to her daily diet with her recent snacks? Provide Virginia with three nutrition-related goals, including specific food suggestions, which will help her to remedy her doctor's concerns.

Crossword Puzzle

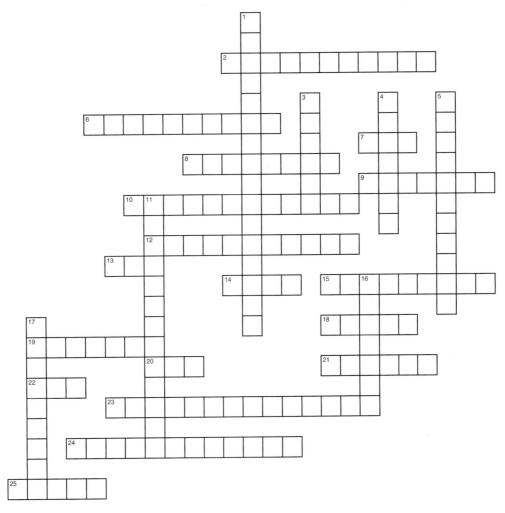

Across

2. when consulting with older athletes about their diet, their medical history, and this must be taken into consideration
6. the key words "balance, variety, and ____" hold true for all athletes regardless of age
7. a great source of protein for vegans
8. alcohol has been noted to stimulate this, which can be a problem if an athlete does not want to gain weight
9. mineral important for young growing athletes
10. the estimated average number of extra calories needed due to pregnancy (2 words)
12. although not technically diabetes, individuals with this condition have higher than normal blood sugar levels
13. type of diabetes in which the pancreas does not secrete adequate amounts of insulin
14. this drink can serve as a healthy snack option for young athletes
15. the growth plate is associated with this part of the typical bone
18. type of vegetarian that eats fish, dairy products, and eggs
19. condition that increases the risk for type 2 diabetes
20. an individual with advanced knowledge and skills for dealing with diabetes mellitus (abbrev.)

21. a B vitamin important for fetal nervous system development
22. alcohol can be readily converted to this in the body
23. an athlete who does not eat any red meat
24. the build-up of intermediate products of fat metabolism causes this clinical condition
25. young athletes should do this throughout the day in order to help meet their dietary needs

Down

1. during pregnancy, adequate hydration is critical to support this physiologic process
3. an athlete over the age of 40 or 50
4. unlike many of the other nutrients we consume, alcohol can be absorbed in this
5. children are at a greater risk for this during exercise than adults (2 words)
11. high blood sugar
16. hormone the stimulates the uptake of blood glucose
17. a common symptom of hypoglycemia

Name: _____   Course Number: _____

Section: _____   Date: _____

CHAPTER 16

Jobs in Sports Nutrition

Working in Sports Nutrition

1. List and describe the three main requirements to become a registered dietitian.

   1. _____

   2. _____

   3. _____

2. Describe the purpose of state licensure of dietitians.

3. Is there licensure of dietitians in the state where you are enrolled in college?

   a. If yes, what organization regulates this licensure? If a dietitian has met the licensure requirements, what credential are they allowed to use?

   b. If no, find a neighboring state that does have licensure for dietitians, and answer the questions above for that state.

4. Find two positions posted on the Internet for sports nutrition jobs. List the professional credentials, education, work experience, and special skills required, or desired, for the position. Identify the skills and credentials you already possess that meet the posting's requirements. Create a plan for how you would obtain the necessary skills and qualifications you do not already have to make you a highly desirable candidate for the job.

You Are the Nutrition Coach

Please read each case study listed below, and answer the associated questions.

1. Katie is a junior exercise science student. She is exploring options for either graduate school or full-time positions after graduation. She knows that she would enjoy doing something related to athletes and sports nutrition. Since Katie is taking only 12 credit hours this semester, she has extra time to pursue opportunities for practical experience in athletics and sports nutrition.

    Question: What opportunities might be available to Katie for practical experience, while she is still working on her exercise science degree?

2. Michael is an RD who has been working in college athletics for 6 years. He has determined that he meets all of the eligibility requirements for taking the CSSD exam. Michael is ready to schedule an exam date, however, he is unsure of where to take the exam, when it is offered, and what materials he should review to prepare for the exam.

    Questions: If Michael lived in your area, where would he go to take the exam? When is the exam offered? What materials should he review before scheduling his exam?

Crossword Puzzle

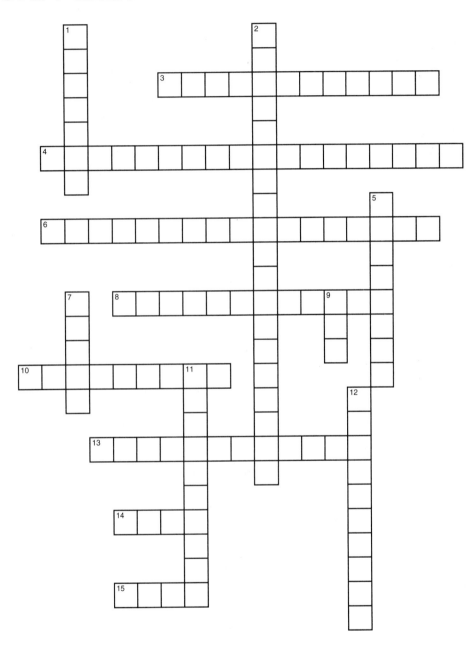

Across

3. way of gaining practical experience in the field of sports nutrition
4. difficult but rewarding job market for a sports dietitian to get into (2 words)
6. one of the most common career choices for sports dietitians (2 words)
8. non-RDs can provide this type of nutritional information (2 words)
10. registration and certification are professionally less restrictive than this
13. anyone that provides dietary information can call themselves this
14. in order to obtain the RD credential, this number of hours of practical experience are required
15. sport-related specialty available to RDs (abbrev.)

Down

1. joining professional state and national organizations can provide an excellent opportunity to _____ with established RDs and nutrition researchers
2. RDs must attain 75 hours of this every 5 years (2 words)
5. the "L" in LD or LDN
7. common non-RD source of nutrition information
9. professional organization for nutrition professionals (abbrev.)
11. the "R" in RD
12. many aspiring RDs do this in order to gain practical experience